Your
Food
FREEDOM

Transforming your
relationship with food

Dimple Thakrar
Bsc (Hons)RD, NLP

2018

Author: Dimple Thakrar
www.nutritionwithdimple.com

Book Layout by Savvy Scripts Publishing
www.savvyscripts.com.au

Photography by briofive.com

Your Food Freedom | Dimple Thakrar. -- 1st ed.
ISBN978-1986120098

DEDICATION

This book is dedicated to the people that inspire me.

To my husband, who has always had faith in my capabilities, even when I have not. You're my absolute rock, I'm nothing without you, and you make me whole. Thank you my love. x

To my daughters Maya and Kiera, my living proof that this works.

To my family – Dad, Mum, Kavita, Rupa, my father-in-law and mother-in-law for believing in me and supporting me. To my mother who was the epitome of fun and laughter and giving unconditional love, while faced with the most challenging conditions. A women so strong and yet so kind, god bless her soul.

To Tony and Sage Robbins for unleashing the power within me to share, grow and impact others by making me realise my truth, my purpose, my calling in life. For teaching me that to give love is so much more fulfilling than to receive. For my awaken, growth and understanding that I was born to serve and contribute. (PS I love it and it makes me feel so alive!)

To my friends and the Robbins family for leading, encouraging and supporting this journey.

To the cosmic universe for bring me the people I needed at the exact time I needed them. Thank you for your pearls of wisdom, your pauses to teach me to catch a breath and smile.

Finally, to my patients – for trusting, believing and taking the leap of faith to Food Freedom with me. Thank you all so much. I'm truly grateful, honoured and privileged to have shared your journey with you.

....

According to the Department of Health it is estimated there are 4 million people in the UK that suffer with eating disorders, though only 1.6 million seek help. The true incidence is very hard to know as we can only guesstimate from the people that seek support. The opposite side to the spectrum is also increasing with 26% of adults in the UK classed as obese. This is soon catching up with our counterparts over the seas in the USA at just under 40%.[37]

My goal is to eradicate eating disorders and distorted eating by helping parents and children live free from food noise in a world of Food Freedom.

I was born to feed both with knowledge, energy and food and so I have decided to contribute...

...50% of the royalties from this book to the Feed-A-Billion Charity - a charity whose sole purpose is to feed people.

Nobody should go hungry in this day and age either through their own choice or unfortunate choices. This charity is so in alignment with my need to feed. I urge you to stay nourished in body, mind, spirit and soul.

With much love this book has been written with my heart and soul. I honour, love and respect each and everyone of you.

Love Dimple x

DISCLAIMER

This book features techniques and information applications that may not be suitable for everyone and is intended only to assist users in their personal nutritional improvement efforts.

Always consult a qualified medical practitioner and or dietitian before starting any new diet, exercise or health programme, or if you have any concerns about your health.

This book is not tailored to individual requirements and is for general information only. Results may vary from individual to individual.

The information in this book should not be taken as professional or medical advice. Do not use the techniques in this book as a substitute for any treatment or medication recommended by a qualified medical professional.

The author, publisher and editors do not accept any responsibility for any adverse effects that may occur due to the use of the information or guidance in this book. If you experience any negative effects, consult a medical professional.

You are urged and advised to seek the advice of a

doctor/physician or dietitian before beginning any exercise and/or nutritional improvement effort or regimen.

This book is intended for use only by healthy adult individuals. The book is not intended for use by minors, pregnant women, or individuals with any type of health condition. Such individuals are specifically warned to seek professional medical advice prior to initiating any form of exercise and/or nutritional improvement effort or regimen.

*To protect the identity of the patient stories in this book, all the names of the patients have been changed.

CONTENTS

CHAPTER ONE

INTRODUCTION

L et me start by introducing myself. My name is Dimple Thakrar. (Yes, Dimple is my real name, not a nickname. My parents thought it would be cute because I was born with dimples and they liked the famous Indian actress Dimple Kapadia.)

Anyway, back to the introduction. I knew at age 13 that I wanted to be a dietitian because I had a keen interest in food, science and people. But it was only when I was in my early 40's, after many years of practice, that I truly understood my calling – the Food Freedom movement, which promotes the ability to take control back from food and have a happy, fulfilling relationship with what you eat.

And that's the basis for this book.

This book is designed to challenge and shift your relationship with food

It will promote self-reflection and ask you to question how your beliefs and values manifest themselves in food. It will challenge your issues with weight and self-worth, and make you work for what you want. It will help define what you're truly striving to achieve and give you a roadmap for getting there. It will address the food noise in your head and aim to give you complete Food Freedom.

If you've failed with diets, are sick of yo-yo dieting and just want inner peace and calm, then this is the book for you.

As with all aspects of personal development, you get what you put in. This book contains mind-set work entwined with evidence-based nutrition information. It's not a recipe book or a nutrition book. It's a book to help you have the most amazing relationship with food, so you can pass on your positivity to the next generation.

A normal, healthy mind, body and soul around food – doesn't that sound nice?

Let me show you how to accept and take

responsibility for changing your habits, so you can move to a place where you're free to choose the foods your body is asking for (the ones that serve your soul, not just your belly).

I promise you this: your family and friends will notice your Food Freedom as you glow with health. I call it the ripple effect.

Are you ready for the ride of your life? The one you've been waiting for? The one that will take you back to your roots of intuitive eating?

I feel privileged to share this journey with you, and I'm grateful for your time and effort. Please sit back, enjoy, think and get nourished.

A FOOTNOTE

I'm passionate about ending the growing madness of eating disorders afflicting today's youth. It's time to stop the epidemic of obesity, orthorexia (fear of unhealthy eating) and more. And an important way to achieve this is by influencing the people that influence young people – especially parents.

Help me help you to model amazing food behaviours and beliefs about body image, weight and health around your children, so we can work together to stop the nutrition media madness.

CHAPTER TWO

A STORY: THE BIRTH OF FOOD FREEDOM

This is the story of how a little girl strived for perfection, nearly killed herself in the process, turned her life around, studied hard and now works to ensure no other woman, girl, man or boy goes through what she did. And to ensure no mother has to endure a child suffering this awful curse – the curse of the eating disorder.

So let me share the biggest secret of my life, a secret not even my children knew about until now.

From when I was five years old, I was a perfectionist – everything had to be just so. I worked hard and was at the top of my class for everything. I went from English being my second language to thinking in English. I went from being the worst reader to the best. I was going to be the best at all costs, and I had a strong and powerful fear within me: the fear of failure. This held me in good stead right though my primary school years, with intellect, willpower and sheer determination getting me through.

Everything was great at this point.

Now I had always been the chubby baby in the family. The cute but rounded middle daughter of 3 girls. Despite being slimmer, neither of my sisters were focused on health and fitness, and they didn't really care what they ate. I, on the other hand, was not going to be the 'fat' one.

My best friend (now my husband, my rock) and my older sister had taken to calling me 'Fats' in a playful, harmless way. Unbeknown to them, it cut like a knife and psychologically triggered something inside of me. I was imperfect, a failure, ugly – and so another challenge rose. I needed to be the thinnest at all cost. I don't blame my husband or my sister for this. Looking back now, what I went through means I can now empathise, help others and perhaps prevent it from happening in the first place. Good comes out of dark times. You have to experience the darkness to seek and realise the light.

And so, aged 11, my rituals for perfection began. I

started running three miles daily, going to the gym after school and doing all the fitness classes I could. I was exercising morning, noon and night. I bought myself a calorie counter bible and I memorised it (great grounding for my life as a dietitian but not helpful for an obsessive child). When I look back I must have been so focused and driven to have managed this level of exercise daily and on such a calorie-controlled diet. I stopped eating all fats and limited my intake to fewer than 1000 kcals a day. I could calculate to the calorie, how much I had consumed, and my aim was to burn all of it exercising. With hindsight it was madness, because we all know that you need energy just to live, and it was really important at that age just to grow!

This continued for at least a year, but probably two. I lost 2 stone, my weight was down to 5 stone, my periods had stopped and my developing breasts had shrunk. But I was still top of the class and I was no longer 'Fats'.

Or was I?

In my mind, I still had 'just a bit' left to lose.

Looking back now, as the mother of two daughters, I shudder to think what my mum and dad must have been going through. I had stopped eating at family functions and parties, and people in the community had started asking if was unwell – they were worried I had some awful disease. I was miserable. Family friends who were doctors started telling my parents I was not normal. My head was so full of guilt, restrictions and striving to achieve the unachievable.

The turning point was when I started to faint at school. I didn't have enough muscle, energy or blood volume to maintain my blood pressure while standing, never mind to support all the sport I was still doing. I had ceased growing, compromised my immune system and stopped my fertility. Now it was affecting my circulation, and the next step would be my heart. If I had to guess, my body fat would have been around 5 to 6%, (normal for this age is anywhere from around 25-30%). So yes, you could say I was motivated enough to achieve anything when I put my mind to it. But at what cost?

Knowing what I know now, I think my obsession was a cry for acceptance and happiness. Like a lot of women, I was seeking this externally – I was looking to change my appearance to be accepted as beautiful, convinced it would lead to my happiness. Little did I know that the more I searched this way, the further away I got.

Authentic happiness was, and always will be, within. Learn to love yourself on the inside, and your external presence will shine.

So what could somebody have told me to prevent that destructive cycle of belief around food, exercise and health? How could my situation have been prevented or turned around sooner? What did I need to know that would have stopped me from permanently damaging my body? Because it didn't have to be that way. So many women have this need to control their food intake and their bodies, to the point where they stop noticing how amazing foods and their bodies actually are. This needs to stop!

We need to find ourselves, trust ourselves and love ourselves. After all, we only have one body. Accept who we are and the rest just happens.

Author and spiritual mentor Rebecca Campbell talks about 'surrendering to your soul.' I would add, 'Surrender to your soul, not your belly.' I will talk about this later in this book.

When I was 13, I decided I needed to find a job that combined all three of my passions: food, science and people. Pharmacy? No, it didn't have food. Doctor? No, I didn't like cutting people up (and I had become a vegetarian). Dietitian? I wasn't sure what it was, so I organised a work placement and spent three days with the local community dietitians. I loved it! I had found my calling. My focus had shifted, and I was learning the truth about food, health and my relationship with my body. I knew I would never model that unhealthy behaviour and language to my future children, especially if I had girls.

It took me years to get to Food Freedom, and if I'm honest, I still have off days (even though they're few and far between). **But it truly is freedom.**

The following chapters contain my lifetime of knowledge around evidence-based nutrition and mind-set, my experiences as a sufferer and a mother, my rigorous training and passion for nutrition and my drive to end food noise and help everyone have Food Freedom. They're about teaching your family how *not* to diet. How to feed souls, not bellies.

For me, the final piece of the jigsaw was understanding the link between **MIND**, **BODY** and **SOUL**

And that's what I now give to you....

CHAPTER THREE

FOOD NOISE AND FOOD FREEDOM DEFINED

You develop your relationship with food over a lifetime. It's formed as you learn to eat as a child and as you develop your knowledge, beliefs and values. That relationship shapes the food choices you make, your feelings and behaviours around food and, ultimately, your perception of your body.

Your relationship with food and your relationship with your body are interdependent. If you can feel good about what you eat, you'll likely feel good about your body. But if you feel bad about what you eat, you're more likely to have negative feelings about your body. So we need to keep that food relationship healthy.

Food noise is the constant, unforgiving, negative and distracting chatter of conversation around food and its impact on your body. These external influences affect food choices and eating behaviour.

FOOD NOISE

Food noise is when food has control. It comes with:

- Distracted or secret eating behaviours

- Mindless eating – no attention to what and how much you're eating

- Guilt-ridden and joyless eating

- Overeating

- Emotionally driven eating

- Periods of food restriction followed by binging

- External influences, such as media, family or friends

Here's an example: You walk past a bakery and find yourself going in and buying cake. You do this, not because you're hungry but because you've been good and you deserve a treat. Or because you're having a bad day and deserve a pick-me-up. Then you find yourself buying three cakes because they were on a special offer (even though you know you don't really want a single cake, never mind three). You eat all three because it would be wasteful not to and feel guilty the whole time you're eating or soon after you've finished.

From this point on, you spend the day obsessing about how you wish you'd never walked past the bakery, or how you wish you'd had the willpower to resist such delicious treats. Then you decide that you may as well eat anything today and start being good tomorrow. And so the food and the external world remain in control while your internal cues remain neglected.

For many patients I've helped through my clinical practice, food noise occupies approximately 90% of their head space. It's time to cut through the noise and take back control – and that's where Food Freedom comes in.

Food Freedom is the freedom to choose what, where, when and how you eat with control, using internal cues rather than external ones.

FOOD FREEDOM

Achieving this has a phenomenal impact on your life. Let's look back at the bakery scenario, this time through the eyes of a person with Food Freedom.

You walk past a bakery and admire the cakes in the window. You ask yourself questions: Do I want one? Am I hungry? Am I just having a bad day? Then you make one of the following choices:

Choice 1: You keep walking

You're not hungry, and even though the cakes are on a special offer, you don't want one because you had a great breakfast and feel full. Thanks, but no thanks for today. You leave the cakes and all thoughts of them in the shop window.

Choice 2: You buy one and save it for later

You notice they have your favourite cake but recognise that you're still full from breakfast. You buy one to eat at your desk during a coffee break when you're a bit peckish. You don't buy three because you won't eat them before they go off, so there isn't any savings in taking up the offer. You eat the cake mindfully when your body is ready for fuel.

If you're satisfied part way through, you don't feel the need to finish it. You enjoy the cake and feel no guilt.

The difference between food noise and Food Freedom isn't whether you eat the cake...

...it's how you eat it

If you're experiencing lots of food noise, the cake has control of your thoughts. If you have Food Freedom, you're in control – you listen to your internal cues, have a rational understanding of your basic physiology and can make the right decision for your mind, body and soul.

When I discuss this with my patients, they often say, 'There's no way normal people do the Food Freedom scenario!' And they're right to be sceptical, because food noise is so ingrained.

This came up in clinic recently with *Ann. Ann worked in the admin department of a bakery, where they had free, fresh cake available every day. She tried to resist and couldn't – she found herself eating at least two cakes a day. Then she would go home and secretly eat packets of sweets when her child had gone to bed. She was convinced she had a sugar addiction.

Within three months of her first consultation, she hadn't even noticed she'd stopped eating the cakes. Not because she was depriving herself, but because she just didn't fancy them. The cakes still arrived daily, but she politely said, 'No, thank you.'

When I asked her when she last said 'yes' to the cakes, she replied, 'Since seeing you, I haven't felt like having one. They just don't appeal to me anymore.' Then I asked her about the secret sweet eating. Her response was, 'You know, I completely forgot I used to do that. What a weird thing to do! I do like sweets and have had them probably three times since I started seeing you, but I've sat down, really enjoyed a few and then left the rest of the packet.'

She had also reached her weight goal. Now she'd done that in the past with other restrictive diets but had never maintained it for longer than a month. When I asked if she could see herself ever going back to that way of eating, her reply was, 'There is no way I can. My body won't let me, and Food Freedom feels too good to stop.'

Then we talked about her food noise levels. At the beginning of her journey, food noise consumed around 95% of her thoughts. This was down to 25%, most of which was health-food awareness. The remaining noise around food was positive and helpful.

I hear variations of this story time and time again, and the positive outcomes all boil down to having control over your response.

This clever formula from Dr. Robert Resnick[1] sums it up:

EVENT + RESPONSE = OUTCOME

You can't always control events or your environment, but if you can change your response you can affect the outcome. Respond as you always do and you'll always get the same outcome. So, if you continue to follow the latest diet, then you'll continue to yo-yo diet and your outcome will be weight gain.

If you choose to do something different and give up the fad diets, you may be surprised at the positive results.

So ask yourself this question: What do you really want? A quick-fix, rapid weight-loss plan that fails after a month (and can even make you fatter)? Or Food Freedom forever?

CHAPTER FOUR

WHAT IS DIETING?

L et's start by just clarifying what 'dieting' means in this context. According to the Oxford English Dictionary, dieting means 'Restricting oneself to small amounts of special kinds of food in order to lose weight.'

Let's break down this definition.

DOES 'RESTRICTING' YOURSELF ACTUALLY WORK?

According to a study of restrained eaters vs. unrestrained eaters, those who hold back on foods are likely to eat more of them.[2] Research also found that restrained eaters responded to high-calorie foods faster than unrestrained eaters.[3]

Think about it for a moment. Imagine I say, 'You're not allowed to have chocolate or a glass of wine (or whatever your pleasure is)?'

You instantly feel like eating/drinking it, right?

You feel a bit naughty, that you're seeking the forbidden fruit, so to speak. You consume it with guilt or in secret, and you over-consume – not for pleasure, but because it's restricted. And you don't enjoy it.

Therein lies the issue: it's not the eating of the treat but the feelings associated with it when you eat it. These lead to feelings of low self-esteem, loss of control and despair, which then perpetuate the need for comfort. And the default source of comfort for many of us, is food. Hence the cycle of diet, restrict, binge, no control, guilt, low self-esteem, failure, emotional binging/mindless eating.

SHOULD YOU FOCUS ON 'SPECIAL KINDS OF FOOD'?

We also need to look at the dictionary definition's use of the phrase 'special kinds of food'. This implies you can't lose weight by eating normal food.

You should want to lose weight to be healthy, but we see images in the media that are far from healthy – and these are the ones people strive to imitate at all costs! When you focus on weight loss instead of health, you get distorted eating and unhealthy relationships with food.[4] And for some high achievers and control freaks, this can be the birth of eating disorders such as orthorexia, a medical condition in which sufferers systematically avoid specific foods they believe to be harmful.

But why should you have to avoid foods to lose weight? And is that behaviour sustainable or healthy? Is this the kind of behaviour we want to be modelling as acceptable for our children?

The confusing mixed messages surrounding food and nutrition all focus on weight rather than health. We're setting our children up to believe that to be socially accepted, they need to look a certain way and/or be on a diet.

CAN DIETING WORK FOR EVERYONE?

Fad dieting often implies that it's one size fits all. But how can the nutritional requirements of a small Indian lady be the same as a tall Dutch lady? It's like saying that a Mini and a Range Rover have the same fuel consumption. It makes no sense. And that leads nicely on to the next chapter on why diets don't work.

CHAPTER FIVE

WHY DIETING DOESN'T WORK

'Many studies show that dieting is a strong predictor of future weight gain.'[5]

H ave you spent years following the latest fad diets? Do you wonder if super foods are actually super (and if they are, how they work)?

Believe me – I know you'll try anything when you're vulnerable and desperate to have control over your eating, your body and your feelings.

A study published in the *American Journal of Public Health*[6] found that how you feel about your body has a higher impact on health and obesity-related disease than your body mass index (BMI – a common measure of weight in relation to height).

Let me explain that a bit more. If you take two women with the same body fat, their health outcomes will vary depending on how they feel about their bodies. And if you take a thin person and an obese person, how they feel about their body has more impact on their health than their BMI. The thinner person could actually have more health risks than the fatter person if they feel stigmatised about their body.

SO THE QUESTION IS: WHY DON'T DIETS WORK?

The answer is simple: a diet only works while you're on it and using all the (often expensive) shakes, powders, bars, pills, tonics or potions. The diet industry is big business – in Europe and the US, annual turnover is in excess of $150 billion (£110 billion).[7] Yes, that's right – billion not million.

The diet industry relies on you failing so you continue to buy the expensive products and memberships. Take a moment to think. Over the years, how much money have you spent on diet stuff? It's frightening. And have you got the body/weight/results you want for the long term?

Now, if your chosen diet asks you to swap foods for shakes or miss out whole food groups like carbs or protein, you're going to lose weight in the short term. Not because carbs are bad for you, but because you've removed a load of calories from your diet.

It's simple maths – if your body needs more calories than you put in, it uses your fat and protein (muscle) stores as fuel, and you lose weight. This is fact, and we'll talk about it in more detail in Chapters 11 to 13.

However, if a diet asks you to remove whole food groups, then it's not balanced – and it will therefore be unsustainable in the long run. Which means ultimately you'll gain weight.

Studies back this up. Weight regain is generally the rule, with 1/3 to 2/3 of the weight lost regained within a year and almost all regained within 5 years. Studies of the long-term outcomes show that at least 1/3 of dieters regain more weight than they lose.[8]

Diets don't work, not just because they're unsustainable, but because the majority don't give you all the nutrients your body needs. And even if they did, they work on the premise of restriction, labelling foods good and bad, punishing for failing and focusing on weight-only outcomes.

You need to address the root causes...

Have you ever felt humiliated or ashamed at weigh-in time?

Dieting is self- destructive because the focus is on negative energy and denial instead of building love for your body and the food you eat.

It should be about health, love and enjoyment of foods.

Food isn't just about nutrition. In fact, I would say nutrition is a very small part of why we eat the foods we do. We're influenced by our upbringing, role models, friends, rituals, behaviours and our personalities around food. Simply addressing a symptom of a very complex issue with a quick-fix diet won't last the long haul.[9]

Instead, we need to understand the reasons why we eat what we do. Start by getting your food facts from a credible source so you have confidence you're eating the right foods to fuel your body. Then think about the behaviours, beliefs and values that shape your identity and purpose around food.

In other words, what do you believe your relationship with food and your body is? Instead of thinking: 'I've always had a problem with my weight.'

Think: 'What values and patterns do I hold around food and my body?' Then we can determine what actions will improve the situation.

Free yourself from food noise because it may be doing more harm than fat

When did you notice yourself shifting away from normal eating (if you can remember what that is) towards this obsession with food and thinness? When did you stop loving your body, if you ever did?

Imagine being able to clear your head of all that food noise and just breathe! Having the head space to do so much more. All the while knowing you're fuelling your body with healthy food, be it a meat-containing, vegetarian or vegan diet. Knowing all the facts and being able to maintain your approach wherever you go – at home, on holiday and eating out.

Imagine a world of guilt-free eating where you love every curve and contour of your gorgeous body. Really, truly feeling blessed for your health, and having your focus shift from weight to a healthy mind, body and soul.

Imagine Food Freedom being the norm for your little ones, where nourishing their bodies means regularly eating a balanced diet and a range of foods.

Think about it – why are many successful dieters still not happy? The stereotype is that thin = happiness and social acceptance, right? We both know that the reality of food, weight, body image and size is very complex, and that dieting is the just the tip of the iceberg. Research suggests that the more we focus on weight alone, the less likely we are to achieve our health and vitality goals.[10]

So let's broaden our focus.

CHAPTER SIX

WHY DO WE DIET?

WHAT DOES DIETING ACTUALLY DO TO YOUR BODY?

Well, by over-restricting your energy intake (the number of calories you eat), you initially lose weight because your body is utilising its fat stores to provide itself with the energy it needs to function.

However, because diets are restrictive and too low in calories, they can prompt a feast-or-famine cycle where periods of restriction are followed by overeating. Over time, this yo-yo dieting pattern causes your metabolic rate to drop as your body prepares for the next famine.[11]

You're not only doing yourself out of calories and vital nutrients, but you're also reducing muscle tissue and gaining extra fat.

Extra fat is storage for the next famine, because the human body is designed to survive against all odds.

This kind of weight cycling also accounts for increased poor health due to inflammation and insulin resistance. It's associated with poor cardiovascular outcomes and a higher risk of death.[12] Plus, evidence suggests that the more you diet, the fatter you get in the long run.[13]

Does that sound familiar? Can you recall how long you've been dieting? Have you achieved and maintained your goal weight?

Take a moment to list how many diets you've done and when you did them. If there's fewer than five, fantastic; if there are more, continue the list on another piece of paper.

Relax, it's not a test – just an exercise in raising your awareness.

DIET NAME	1	2	3	4	5
YEAR					
HOW YOU FELT A YEAR AFTER THE DIET					
TOTAL COST OF THE DIET					

Do you feel happy? Successful? Sad? Despairing? Think about who was in control - you or the diet?

Now let's look at your current (or most recent) diet. How much did you weigh when you started, how much do you weigh now and what's the difference between the figures?

STARTING WEIGHT: ___
MINUS
CURRENT WEIGHT: ____
EQUALS
WEIGHT LOSS SO FAR: _____

Is it where you want to be? Are you happy with your current body? Have you ever seen yourself the size you're striving for in your mind's eye?

I bet the answer to this is no. Why? Because you're focusing on trying to lose weight and not on the end goal of being healthy and comfortable in your amazing body.

When you set your SATNAV to weight loss, guess what happens? You're always trying but you never achieve the actual goal – which is happy mind, body and soul.

It's time to stop spending money on quick-fix diets that make you fat.

THE **TEN** FOOD COMMANDMENTS

1. Stop dieting and restraining

2. Start living

3. Start loving your food and body

4. Food is for pleasure

5. Food is to share love

6. Food is memory-making

7. Food is for nourishment

8. Food is fuel for performance in mind, body and soul

9. Understand why we need food

10. Respect the fuel and it will respect you

Why are we bombarded with the latest celebrity diet? How have we become a nation of obsessive dieters? Why do we see these diet-culture messages everywhere? Why is it acceptable to be inundated with damaging messages from unqualified people?

Social media has made a massive positive impact on our lives, but it's a double- edged sword because it makes it hard to tell what information is accurate and science-based. It's easy to read someone's opinion online and think it's fact.

This era of fast information and fast results has led us to a false sense that everything should be fast, free and easy. At least that's what the adverts say...Weight loss, the perfect body – get it today with minimal effort! (And of course there's a bit of air-brushing for good measure. Perfection and air-brushing have become so normalised that my 12-year-old daughter had to write an essay on it for school!)

With all this social pressure, it's obvious why women and men, girls and boys now try to achieve unrealistic and unhealthy body goals by unscientific and possibly dangerous methods.

We no longer need to put our bodies through fads and famine. We just need to make peace with our bodies and become in tune with them.

CHAPTER SEVEN

YOU WOULDN'T GO TO A BUTCHER FOR SURGERY...

...WOULD YOU?

A t a basic level, both butchers and surgeons cut meat. So why wouldn't you go to a butcher for surgery?

As you recoil at the question, consider this – it's actually the same as going to an unqualified 'guru' for nutrition advice.

WHAT IS A DIETITIAN?

Unlike the people hawking fad diets, dietitians aren't trained in marketing and generally shy away from promoting themselves.

Being a dietitian is a bit like being a food doctor.

In the UK, 'dietitian' is a protected title. That means you can only call yourself a dietitian if you have completed a 4 ½- year undergraduate degree or a post-graduate degree in dietetics. We can only work and advise on evidence-based nutrition because we're bound by a code of conduct, very much like doctors.

Most dietitians are members of a professional association – in Britain it's the British Dietetic Association (BDA), which holds lists of independent and NHS dietitians in your area. All dietitians must be registered with a governing council – this is standard practice for most health professionals, and the governing body makes sure they have the right qualifications. In the UK, it's the Health Care Professional Council. I must renew my registration every two years and prove I'm up to date with all the latest evidence and science. Check me out before you read any further – it's always good practice to verify credentials before you get advice from anybody.

HOW IS A DIETITIAN DIFFERENT TO A NUTRITIONIST?

'Nutritionist' also isn't a protected title in the UK, so anybody can call themselves a nutritionist whether they have done a two-week course or a degree. And it can be hard to tell who's done the degree and who's done a free online course. Also, their training only includes working with people who are well, not people with illnesses such as diabetes, heart disease or cancer. Dietitians train to work with both types of people. If you want to see a specialist about your diet (and by that, I mean the food and drink you eat normally, not in the sense of 'being on a diet'), check they have the right credentials for your needs.

If you have no medical issues and you know the nutritionist sitting in front of you is suitably qualified, then go ahead. But if you have medical issues like Coeliac Disease, medically diagnosed intolerances or Irritable Bowel Syndrome, for example, you're best off seeking help from a dietitian.

Don't get me wrong – there are some amazing nutritionists out there. But there are also some who give advice that's not been proven to be safe. So why take very harmful nutrition advice from celebs, bloggers or vloggers who are just telling you their story – not science and not something that's necessarily safe for you?

...it's like trusting a butcher to operate on you...

THE BIRTH OF FOOD FREEDOM

I became a dietitian in 1995 and worked my way up through the NHS. I started out helping patients with Diabetes, weight loss and Heart Disease and then did research into Coeliac Disease (an auto-immune disease that causes gluten intolerance). Then, for 15 years, I worked with people suffering from neurological problems.

You might be wondering what my CV has to do with you and this book. Well, I've always loved my work, but after raising my two girls (now 18 and 12), I felt my purpose wasn't being fulfilled. I had more to give. But what was it?

Alongside my NHS work, five years ago I started my private practice and completed a neurolinguistic programming (NLP) course. This course gave me the tools to identify my purpose in life.

It hit me like a bolt of lightning.

One day, when my daughters were arguing over who had the most of their five a day (that's at least five fruit and veg a day). I had invested so much time and energy into raising them to have an amazingly healthy relationship with food and their bodies. Now they were competing over fruit and veg intake and asked questions like 'Is this meal balanced?' and 'Where are my protein and carbs?' There were no conversations about good and bad foods or cutting out foods because they didn't want to get fat.

The language, the relationship they had with food was so positive, and their focus wasn't on being thin but on being healthy. My girls had Food Freedom naturally! They had no food noise in their heads – just room to grow, develop, learn and focus on being the best they could be. And I had taught them that!

It suddenly dawned on me that the years of consistently teaching them the basics of nutrition, teaching them to use language around health and not weight, to praise and love every single part of their beautiful bodies inside and out, to role model those behaviours as the norm – it had paid off. I was so proud. And I started to think about how exactly I did it.

I soon noticed that I was using the same approach and messages with my private patients. What sounded normal to me and my family wasn't normal for everyone else. And my purpose was born. My soul was finally being heard, and my calling was being met. The concept of Food Freedom was born.

My mission was now Food Freedom for all, be it learned or modelled. I wanted to empower people to have an amazingly healthy relationship with food and their bodies – for life.

I wanted to convey simple, important nutrition messages, particularly to young women and mothers, so they had a way to achieve Food Freedom in their everyday lives. This, in turn, would impact their children, who would have the same healthy relationship my girls enjoy. They'd be confident and healthy, without the same burden of societal expectations and yo-yo dieting. By giving parents and teachers Food Freedom, the benefits would cascade down to the little people.

What could be a more rewarding purpose? God, I love my job.

Over the years, I've helped many people develop this positive relationship with food and gain control of their eating – for many, it was the first time they'd achieved this. The initial process generally takes just three sessions over four weeks. We undo all the harmful nutrition information and food noise, often from unqualified people, and set the story straight with sound science and common sense. We all have grandmas and grandads who ate everything and lived full, long and diet-free lives, don't we? The common-sense element has gone! How can a diet of eating only grapefruit or just drinking juice give you all the nutrients your body needs over the long term?

'Well, how do I do it?' I hear you ask.

This is what I will share with you over the next few chapters. I'll start by going through the basic nutrient groups, giving a simple overview of what each one does for you. Then I'll explain how you change your relationship with these foods so they have a more positive impact on you and your body.

CHAPTER EIGHT

SLAVE TO THE SCALES

- Do you weigh yourself more than once a day?

- Do the scales decide how your day is going to pan out?

- Do they determine what, where and how you're going to eat that day?

If the answer to these questions is yes, then you're definitely a slave to your scales.

I once asked these same three questions as part of a seminar I gave to a group of ladies. It was thought-provoking, because many of them hadn't realised that this behaviour had become normal for them. It was almost as if they were on autopilot when they stood on the scales every morning and night. The scales dictated how they ate, breathed, lived and felt. Imagine coming to the realisation that a small machine has so much control?

Not only had I raised their awareness of the behaviour, but they also recognised how that behaviour affected their children. One lady remembered her child asking why she measured her feet daily. Had she expected them to grow? When I asked the ladies how this realisation made them feel, many were alarmed at the control those numbers had over them, and at the behaviour they were normalising.

Before we go into the roadmap to achieving Food Freedom, it's important to address this issue of the scales, because you need to have realistic goals. Many people set unattainable weight goals that aren't authentic to their true self. And that contributes to the yo-yo dieting and self-perpetuating negativity.

Your actual goal should be to be in love with yourself and your body. When you achieve this, you end up reducing comfort eating, binging, starvation and the physical and emotional turbulence of the dieting roller coaster.

The evidence suggests that focusing on weight

stigma and feeling bad about your body actually makes you eat more.[14] In one study of 2,944 people, researchers found that the more people focused on weight over wellbeing and vitality, the more weight they gained and the larger their waists became.[15]

In another study, 'overweight' and 'normal'-weight women were showed one of two videos - one stigmatised weight and the other had neutral content. The women who watched the stigmatising video ate more than the ones who watched the neutral one. In the case of the 'overweight' women, it was three times as many calories.[16]

So, what does this all mean? The stigma and negative stimulation caused women to eat more, irrespective of their weight.

Do you recognise this pattern in yourself? Think about how you feel when you weigh yourself or somebody makes a comment about your weight. If the numbers are higher than you'd like or if the comment is negative, how does it affect you?

HOW I FREED MYSELF FROM THE SCALES

I often get asked what I weigh and how I consistently remain the same weight while still having fun and a social life.

When I was a slave to the scales, if I saw the number going up I would think, 'Sod it' and go eat – because I may as well since I'd put weight on anyway! If the number went down, I was motivated to continue and not overeat. Can you relate to this feeling? Who has the control in this situation? The scales, or you?

I decided that weighing myself was counter-productive, and that as long as my jeans fit I was fine. I'm probably the heaviest I've ever been but the smallest size because I do a lot of weight lifting. As we all know, muscle weighs more than fat. Either way, I have no idea about my weight or percentage body fat, nor do I care. As long as I feel good, I have control. I'm not a slave to the scales anymore. And that's worth celebrating.

In my experience, when you focus on your true self, you can end up being the size and weight you should actually be. Now this may not be your ideal number, but if you're happy and feel good about yourself, you often get complimented on your appearance – and this makes you feel more amazing than being super skinny and miserable. And remember the research we discussed in Chapters 5 and 6? It suggests that you may actually be better as a fit, heavier person than as a thin person.

*So, don't focus on weight loss –
see it as a by-product of having
a positive relationship with your
food and your body.*

I know this can sound alien because it's so different
to what you've always done and how you've always
thought. But if you continue to do what you've always
done, you'll struggle to get a different result. So it's
time to take a leap of faith. After all, what do you
have to lose?

DIMPLE'S FOUR RULES FOR ESCAPING SCALE SLAVERY

1. If weighing yourself makes you feel bad, don't do it. It's pointless because you'll just feel worse and eat more.

2. Weighing yourself more than once a week is pointless. Try to stick to weighing yourself once a month. Your weight can fluctuate by a few kilograms due to water and hormones.

3. Use other measures of your success, like how your jeans fit and how you feel. Have you noticed that when you're having a good day, you feel good, look good and people comment (no matter what your size/weight is)? You're the only one who cares about the number.

4. Take 100% responsibility for your actions. The scales aren't in control, you are!

CHAPTER NINE

SET THE SATNAV

THIS CHAPTER IS ALL ABOUT SETTING YOUR GOALS.

Naturally, all my weight-loss patients come to me wanting to lose weight. And they're very surprised when I say I don't weigh people or focus on weight. After all, how else will we know if the diet is working? Then we talk about their past diets and how the only goal has been weight loss (no matter what). The conclusion is always that past diets haven't worked (otherwise they wouldn't be in my office).

Setting the SATNAV to your true destination will get you to the right place

What are you true goals? How do you shift focus? These are all questions I get asked regularly, so let's have a look at them.

The key is to hone in on the right goal. So, if you say 'I'm big boned,' or 'I've always been fat,' or 'I will never stop eating sugar,' your internal SATNAV will set itself to stay on that mental pathway. Your self-limiting beliefs and visualisations will guide your behaviours to maintain your body as it is.

So why haven't you achieved your ideal body or weight? Because you haven't actually set your SATNAV to it. You still visualise yourself as a sugar addict or as a big- boned person. You stay focused on your current destination.

Here's what I mean. Imagine it's January and you've made a New Year's resolution to lose weight. You tell yourself that this is the year you're going to do it. But in the back of your mind, you know you'll be thinking the same next year after having tried this year's fad/celeb diets.

How do you visualise yourself? Is it the size and shape you are or the size and shape you want to be? In your mind's eye, do you see yourself as a thin or fat person? Do you ever wonder how thin people stay thin? Or how they stay motivated to go to the gym and choose healthy foods?

Before we do anything in life, we have to visualise ourselves doing it. Going to work or going to the gym, we preview it in our heads first to prepare ourselves mentally.

In other words, you set your SATNAV for it. And you have to do the same for your body goals. It's important that you're truly honest with yourself when you do this. If you want a six-pack and know you can incorporate the necessary work into your schedule, then great. But you won't achieve it if there's a little voice in your head saying, 'No, that's not actually going to happen – you're just kidding yourself.' It's great to have goals that challenge you, but only if you're being true and authentic to yourself.

It's time to ask yourself what you really want? Is it weight loss – or is it freedom from dieting, with complete control over your eating? Many of my patients feel their lives are dictated by food noise. The food noise is dominant so the SATNAV sets itself to focus on it, thereby influencing behaviour, feelings and emotions and resulting in the undesired body.

Here's an example of what I mean. I asked *Suzy about her goals and she immediately showed me a photo of a 6-foot fitness model in a bikini. Suzy ran a super successful business and barely made time to eat, let alone work out daily.

'How often do you think that model spends maintaining that physique?' I asked her. 'Hours every day, I should think,' my patient replied.

In admitting that, Suzy internalised what she'd have to sacrifice (her business) to achieve that goal. During that moment of true authenticity, she realised that her weight wasn't actually her main goal – her goal was to manage her anger and lift her mood. Yes, she would like to be thinner as a by-product, but she was most excited when she talked about being happy, not snapping at her staff or feeling frustrated all the time. Just a few months later Suzy, has reorganised and reallocated her work load and now does the work she loves to do. All because she started to fuel that beautiful body and mind and was able to think clearly. She lost the 8 lbs she wanted with very little effort and loving what she eats and does for a living. No hangry or anger, just in complete feminine flow.

HOW TO SET YOUR SATNAV AND REACH THE RIGHT DESTINATION

You start by creating a standard for yourself that's a must-have, not a should-have. This is who you are, not the 'new you' but YOU. The person who wears the clothes you want to wear, the person who lives a healthy life.

If you need help defining your standard because you're not what you want to be, ask your soul: it's dying to tell you. You may have been suppressing it with food for many years as you fed your belly instead, but it's desperate to be heard.

'How do I ask my soul?' you're wondering. Well, meditation helps you dampen the noise that blocks you hearing your soul. It helps you understand what it is your soul truly wants. You'll be amazed at what comes out. Try it and see what message you hear. It may be that you're happy at this weight and just need to get fitter. Or that you really want to try a new sport. Or that dancing is actually your passion. Once you've discovered what your soul has known all along, you can visualise the true you. And don't be surprised at what you see. This is your identity. It's who you are. It's your new higher standard.

Once you have that standard, you can think about the rituals and behaviours you need to maintain yourself at that standard. It takes conscious effort to begin with, but your need to be that person is so strong and has such pull that the rituals become a necessity, a way of life. So, healthy eating or going to the gym becomes the same as brushing your teeth – an intrinsic part of your day.

Step 1: Decide who you are and define your identity by meditating and asking your soul

Visualise that person – it's your destination. It needs to be done with truth, honesty and authenticity. I'm 5 feet 2½ inches (the ½ inch matters when you're a perfect small package). If I visualise a 6-foot blond as my ultimate goal, it's a pointless exercise. You have to be honest to know what you really want in your heart.

When the true you is revealed, pay attention to the picture. Is it in colour or black and white? Is it still or moving? What are you doing? Who are you with? What are you wearing? Describe your clothes and how you feel in them. What are other people saying around you? What are their expressions? What are your facial expressions? Are you smiling? How are you feeling? How do others make you feel? Describe what you can hear, feel, smell and taste.

Really take a moment to get into this zone. When you're there, absolutely revel in it. Then, when you're really feeling in the moment, ask yourself what animal represents this feeling.

Allow the animal to plop. Don't be surprised by what arrives. I've heard all sorts, from lions to stallions to glam dogs! This is a symbol of how you feel in that moment. Hold on to that image, so that when you're feeling lost you can use it to guide your SATNAV back to your destination. It's a tool you can use to help you keep on track. It comes from your soul – a place that feels good and right, a place of inner peace and comfort.

Step 2: Think about what habits and Rituals are stopping you from being that true authentic person

Starting from that place of inner peace, list the things you do daily that prevent you being that person/animal? What's holding you back from being a glam dog? It might be taking the lift, or oversleeping so you don't have time for that walk. You must figure these out and write them down.

Step 3: Write down the rituals/behaviours you're going to commit to daily and forever

Think about how you can change the behaviours in Step 2 to achieve your animal and be that standard of person, that identity your soul has been calling you to be.

To achieve this standard, you'll need to put in effort on a consistent, daily basis. You need to develop habits. So, they could be eating healthily most of the time or going to the gym four times a week. The work becomes linked with your identity and how you honestly visualise yourself – so the rituals, habits and behaviours become part of your life.

It's not: 'Maybe I'll go to the gym today,' or 'I'll have a day off and eat rubbish.' It's: 'I will go to the gym,' and 'I will eat healthily.' It's a complete shift in mind-set. Being the body shape you visualise for yourself isn't an option but a must-have, and so the rituals aren't an option either. But you got to be honest, I would love to be 5ft 7inches and long legged, but it isn't going to happen and I am just kidding myself at 5ft 2inches. I am a perfectly formed curvy, small package of beauty. Speak the truth and be true to yourself and love every curve, because that is who you are – beautiful from the inside out.

Step 4: List the reasons to maintain that person, that animal

You have your destination and you have your roadmap. To maintain the habits and behaviours, you need to be clear on the reasons why you're doing this. List what you gain by doing the rituals daily to maintain your animal. For some, it's longevity. For others, it's good health to play with grandchildren. Or avoiding illness. Or happiness, control, inner peace, Food Freedom and a reduction in food noise.

Remember, Muhammad Ali didn't become the greatest by not training, or eating rubbish food. He became the greatest by consistently putting in the work, telling himself he was the greatest and visualising himself as such. So, when he trained (which was a non-negotiable daily ritual, by the way), he trained like a champion. Now, go find your inner champion and train like it.

Show up and do what it takes to be that person, knowing why and what you will gain from doing so.

BUT WHAT ABOUT THE OFF DAYS? HOW TO COME UNSTUCK

'Habit-based interventions show promising results in sustaining behaviour change.'[17]

What about the days when you feel emotional and all you want to do is eat? This is when you have to learn to change 'state'. State is the power of your mind, it's how you feel emotionally and it governs whether you're paralysed or moved to take action.

A controlled, uncomfortable state often makes us act, and this can be positive or negative. The key is the uncomfortableness.

There's a school of thought that says when you're on the edge of your comfort zone and pushed just outside it (but not in panic), you're more likely to change. *(See the fantastic diagram below.)*

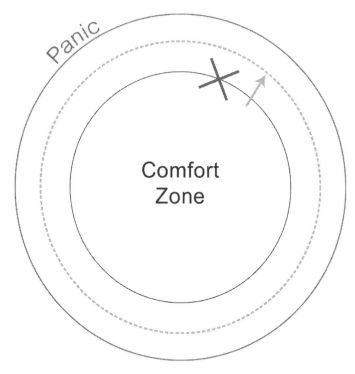

You see, you need your state to be uncomfortable in order for you to want to make changes. The trick is not to be pushed into panic mode, so you're paralysed at best and destructive at worst. An example of panic-mode behaviour is emotional overeating – you feel so out of control that your behaviour becomes destructive and irrational.

Sound familiar? Let's face it if we weren't uncomfortable why would we change, we would be very comfortable and not bother?

If you can think of a time when you were upset with yourselves for binging or letting your self down and you were uncomfortable, you said "No more! I am not doing this again". That is when you were on the edge of your comfort zone (blue cross) and you changed, and that behaviour, be it exercising or stopping eating that particular food or less of it, became the norm. Your comfort zone grew (green line). That is how we grow and make long- lasting behaviour changes. We need to grow over comfort zones by pushing ourselves to the edge and feeling a little uncomfortable.

Let's think about how we can produce a state that moves us towards our goals. Shifting your state must involve mind, body and soul because they're linked. This next technique is something I learned from listening to and using Tony Robbins' teachings, and I therefore respectfully attribute this to him.

1. Move your physical state

Notice your posture when you feel sad or are emotionally eating. What's it like? Is your head held high? Are you smiling? Are you taking controlled deep breaths? Hell no. Your head is stooped and you can barely smile.

First you have to break the pattern and move. Get out of your chair and walk. Hold your head high. Put on music that makes you feel good, dance and sing. You may not feel like it and it will feel weird at first, but it beats eating when you don't want to eat (and it's impossible to feel sad when you're singing your favourite up-beat song).

2. Control the mental talk

Be aware of the words you keep replaying in your head. 'I'm big boned and I'm always going to be fat.' Change the record, because that record keeps those self- limiting beliefs larger than life.

What's your mental mantra? What's your new story? Use your visualisation. Muhammad Ali's was 'I'm the greatest.' He believed he was the greatest and he was. His mental mantra dictated his beliefs. What's your mantra? What are your positive affirmations? Repeat them over and over again. Make signs and put them in places you see every day. Make them your screensaver. For example, if your visualisation is you wearing an amazing red dress, your mantra could be, 'I look and feel amazing in that red dress.' Believe it's possible and it will be. Act as if it's already achieved. You're wearing and feeling amazing in the red dress.

3. Shift your emotional state

Have you ever tried feeling sad in a state of gratitude? It's impossible to feel sad when you're feeling grateful for the world and your life. Shifting emotional state is as simple as pausing and noticing what you're grateful for.

Make a list of three things you're grateful for and really feel your sense of gratitude. Close your eyes and visualise the three things – note the sounds, smells, colours, movements and feelings of joy. It could be something as simple as the birds singing or the bluebells starting to open.

Often, it's the simplest things that make us most grateful and give us the greatest sense of joy. Now, think about the thing that made you emotionally eat before? Does it feel as strong now?

Practising these techniques when you're in a stuck position engages your mind, body and soul to help you shift.

There's a growing body of research demonstrating that knowledge alone doesn't empower and facilitate long-term change. Instead, knowledge with beliefs and strategies on how to achieve change is super powerful in improving some health areas and maintaining results.

An example of this is a study of people with Type 2 Diabetes. Half were treated with an empowerment programme based on behaviour change and the other half received conventional treatment. The group with the empowerment programme showed significantly more improvement in their diabetic control than the group without it.[18]

'Knowledge, in and of itself, does not lead to behaviour change; however, knowledge and health beliefs are linked to engagement in self-regulation.'[19]

How many times has your doctor asked you to stop smoking or lose weight or change your lifestyle – and told you all the reasons why? And you walk out of the consultation thinking, 'Whatever, he doesn't understand my life.' Or 'It's easy for him to say – he doesn't have the stresses that I have.' Nothing changes, you go back the following year and the cycle repeats itself.

You have the knowledge so why don't you just do it?

Well, until you believe it's important, until you realise the pain or benefit you get from the change, nothing changes. Knowledge alone doesn't prompt action – you need the right information, the belief it's important, the reasons why and the steps you're going to take to make the changes happen in your life.

CHAPTER TEN

THE BAR'S OPEN - ANYONE FOR WATER?

The next few chapters give you clear, easy-to-follow, evidence-based nutrition messages. They set the record straight amidst all the 'facts' you see from media, celebs, social media, friends and family. Finally, practical and trustworthy nutrition! Enjoy.

Water is the most abused and undervalued nutrient, yet it makes up between 60 and 70% of our bodies. Imagine you wanted to bake a cake and you only used eggs and sugar. You would have a flat, sugary mess, at best.

Yet daily I see people who don't even consider that a lack of water in their diet may be contributing to symptoms like fatigue, constipation, headaches, low mood and bloating. There are reams of research on this,[20] and yet people don't realise the impact dehydration (even a mild 1 to 3%) can have on the body.

And when I say body, I mean your head, too. If the brain is even mildly dehydrated, it can lead to low mood, increased anxiety, poor memory and headaches. There are even studies where people who drink water before meals lost 44% more weight over 12 weeks than those who didn't.[21] Other studies have put this down to feeling fuller while eating, and therefore eating less.[22]

Now, you know I'm not about weight loss – I'm about loving who you are and the body you have. But surely this is enough evidence and common sense for you to stop spending money on expensive coffees, energy drinks, headache tablets, laxatives or magic pills that give you an energy boost, and just drink more of the free stuff.

Let me tell you about *Joleen. She was a 30-something mum of two young children. At the beginning of her marriage, before the children, a family tragedy meant she had to help care for a relative. I'm talking helping them go from intensive care and several operations to good health.

It was years of rehab. Joleen was strong and she managed, but it left her dependant on antidepressants due to the stress of the constant caring, the physical toll of daily trips to the hospital and the emotional uncertainty of whether the loved one would survive.

Not only did this impact her mental wellbeing, but it affected her physically as well, and she battled with her weight. As she yo-yo dieted, her weight increased and decreased. After a few years and two children, she was a stone heavier than she needed to be. Now this may not sound like much, but at 5 feet 1 inch, a stone was a lot of extra to carry. And besides the weight, she was unhappy with the way she looked and how her clothes fit.

Joleen came to me for help. Three months and five sessions later, she had lost her weight despite having Christmas, two birthday parties and a family holiday. Her symptoms of constipation, bloating and tiredness had disappeared. She was feeling totally unstoppable. She even contacted her doctor about reducing her antidepressants, and felt amazing when she did.

So far, so good. But months later, she contacted me because her symptoms of bloating, fluid retention, weight gain and low mood had returned, and she was worried she might have developed a food intolerance. I asked a few questions. She was still following the Food Freedom model but had stopped drinking as much water as recommended. She had increased her exercise and reduced her water intake.

Double whammy! Her body had started to retain water because it wasn't getting enough, a bit like camels do; she was gaining water weight and dehydrating her body and brain at the same time.

I asked her to take note of how much she was drinking and assess for herself if it was enough. Guess what she realised that by increasing her intake by two extra glasses a day all her pain, bloating and uncomfortableness disappeared. How often do you think you are drinking plenty and then realise when you stop and calculate that you aren't? It happens to me too from time to time.

As long as you are aware of your bodies signals for when things aren't quiet right and you listen and take action, you will always be in balance with your bodies needs.

HOW MUCH WATER SHOULD YOU DRINK?

A basic guide is 30 to 35ml per kilogram of body weight. So if you weigh 60kg, for example, your requirement is 1,800ml to 2,100ml.

However, you need to check what your urine is like. If it's dark and smelly, then you need more water. If you're constipated and eat at least five servings of fruit or veg a day, then you need more. If you're retaining fluid in your arms or legs, you probably need more. Ditto if your clothes feel tight around the waist and you have no other medical conditions like heart, liver or kidney disease.

If after drinking more water (a minimum of 8 x 8oz glasses a day) you're still having symptoms of constipation, dark urine or oedema/fluid retention, then you may need to see your doctor.

CHAPTER ELEVEN

CARBOHYDRATES: THE BAD BOYS... ...(NOT)

Recently, a trainer at a gym described carbohydrates as 'devil food.' She went on to tell me that she never eats bread but often binges on muffins and cakes!

Carbs have had some very bad press recently, resulting in people becoming confused (like this trainer, who would rather avoid a good energy source for a higher calorie, fat and sugar food).

Before I start with the science behind carbohydrates, let me tell you about Jody. Jody was a very active 50 year old who ran half marathons and cycled for fun at the weekends. She had always been a fit, healthy and slim lady, taking care of her body with healthy, balanced eating and regular exercise. She never struggled with her weight and was a slender size 10 (a 6 in US sizing). She loved her body and her life, and was a fun, outgoing businesswoman. She was a single parent raising her beautiful daughter. She often contributed to charities by doing challenges, which gave her physical goals and fulfilled her need to give back to society. She had it all – the fabulous body, seemingly eating what she wanted, including carbs with every meal, and loving life as a successful and independent woman. So you're probably wondering why she sought me out, right?

Well, her brother was getting married and she thought, 'Wouldn't it be great to get into a size 8 dress? How hard could it be to drop a dress size?'

So, she started seeing a qualified physiotherapist and she set about her goal. She decided to cut out carbs because the media and fitness industry were promoting this approach to rapid weight loss. The physiotherapist was good at training but also supported her quick weight loss with this nutritional advice. *(Remember Chapter 7 about going to the butcher for surgery?)*

Now Jody was super driven, as you can imagine, and so was focused on achieving her goal no matter what. She trained to the max and followed a low-carb, high-protein diet with plenty of veg and salad. You would think, 'Great! She's bound to lose weight and improve her performance, getting stronger, leaner and fitter. Right?' Wrong!

She got bigger, stored more fat, and her running times got slower. She became fatigued and constipated, and the more she tried the more these symptoms persisted. To top it off, she had developed massive sugar cravings, which she had never experienced before. She even went to her doctor and got her blood tested for disease or deficiency, but the tests showed nothing. Jody, the doctor and the physiotherapist were baffled. She had gone from a gorgeous, lean size 10 to a fatter size 14, and was feeling unhappy and low in mood. She hated the way she looked, and the more she dieted, the bigger and wobblier she got. Her physiotherapist had written another letter to her doctor urgently requesting a medical review for fear of some underlying disease.

At this point she came to me, blaming all this on the menopause. Within 2 weeks of following my advice, eating balanced meals and reintroducing carbohydrates, her fatigue disappeared, sugar cravings stopped, clothing felt looser and her performance had measurably improved. She felt amazing! On returning for her third session just 4 weeks later, she reported taking 9 minutes off her half marathon time. Her physiotherapist could not believe her recovery. Now, 6 months in, she's back to her healthy size 10, gone through the menopause – and feeling sexier than ever!

Here's the science behind what happened with Jody, so you can make informed choices in your own life.

SIMPLE SUGARS

Carbohydrates are split into two – simple sugars and complex carbs (or starches).

Let's start with the simple sugars, as they're the easiest and everyone loves to eat them. These are the carbs found in sweet things – any white, brown, caster or icing sugar. They're the sugars found in cakes, biscuits, sweets and desserts. Then there are the sugars people think are healthier, but I'm sorry to say are still sugars and work in our bodies in exactly the same way, like honey, syrup, molasses and fructose.

All simple sugars break down in the body to the same number of calories (4 kcals per gram). Because they taste sweet and are concentrated, you're more likely to overindulge on them. Also, they tend to be combined with high-fat foods like cakes and biscuits, which give you very few other nutrients. For example, a 5g teaspoon of sugar gives you 20 kcals. A

5g teaspoon of honey gives you 50 kcals. So if you're trying to lose weight, simple sugars aren't the best way to get all your calories because they don't give you any other benefits or nutrients. They're empty calories. No vitamins, minerals, essential fatty acids – nothing.

WHAT HAPPENS WHEN WE EAT THESE TYPES OF FOOD?

Here's the science bit. When you eat or drink something high in simple sugar, it needs very little digestion. Some of it is absorbed into your bloodstream from your mouth before it even hits your stomach. This means the sugar from your mouth moves into your blood almost immediately, raising your blood sugar very quickly. This is sometimes called a sugar rush.

Now, the closer the food is to sugar in its natural form, the quicker it's absorbed and the less digestion is required. Sugary drinks move very quickly from the stomach into the blood, whereas a muffin may take longer because the sugar is wrapped with flour and fat. The stomach has to work on all those components to release the simple sugar into the bloodstream, but it's still a relatively fast process, taking around 20 minutes depending on the portion size and what else is in your stomach. Once the sugar hits the blood, it boosts your blood sugar levels and is then very quickly transported to all the other parts of the body for energy. Once it reaches these parts - like the brain, heart, lungs, muscles and other organs - your blood sugar levels fall.

So to recap: the simple sugars are rapidly absorbed into the blood, which acts as a motorway system moving the sugar to where it's needed. The organs need that sugar as a fuel source to survive, to keep us ticking over. So why does a vital nutrient like simple sugar get such bad press? And why are we asked to reduce our sugar intake?

Well, we live in a society with affluent and sedentary lifestyles, were food is plentiful and activity isn't. We're able to get fuel for our organs from other sources, so this quick release but suddenly plummeting source leads to us to overeat, because high sugar foods taste good. This means we end up putting too much fuel in the tank and not burning it off. The extra that's overeaten is stored in the body as – guess what? You got it! Fat.

The idea that sugar turns to fat isn't actually true. Any extra energy we eat, whether it comes from fat, sugar, protein or complex carbohydrates, is stored as fat if it's not burned off. Because, in the days of feast and famine, this was our body's way of preparing for the famine. But in this day and age, the famine never comes!

FREE VS. INTRINSIC SUGARS

'Free sugars are those added to food or those naturally present in honey, syrups and unsweetened fruit juices, but exclude lactose in milk and milk products.'[23]

Free sugars are found freely in food. It's sugar as we know it – the sugar in cakes, biscuits and drinks. These sugars are absorbed very quickly by the body, often through the mouth especially if in liquid form. These sugars cause the most harm to teeth and can be easily overeaten, contributing to obesity and childhood diabetes.

The Scientific Advisory Committee on Nutrition (SACN) is an independent group that provides guidance to the government. It gives us the following recommendations:[24]

- 19g or 5 sugar cubes for children aged 4 to 6
- 24g or 6 sugar cubes for children aged 7 to 10
- 30g or 7 sugar cubes for children 11 years and over, based on average population diets

This equates to no more than 5% of our total calories coming from free sugars. Current consumption equates to 14 to 15%, with fizzy drinks consumption at its highest in teenagers. So sugar is a biggie when it comes to weight gain (but I think we all knew that).

Sugar found in whole fruit and unflavoured natural milk is classed as an intrinsic sugar – sugar locked within the natural structure of the food. Intrinsic sugars don't have the same harmful effect on teeth and health as free sugars.

Here's an example. A chocolate biscuit is equivalent to an apple in terms of calories. Here's the breakdown:

Chocolate biscuit	Small apple
86 kcals	78 kcals
5.1 g of sugar	15 g sugar
4.1 g fat	0 g fat

I know what you're thinking – the apple has three times more sugar than the biscuit. However, for that sugar and calorie content, the apple is going to take you longer to eat because it's high in soluble fibre. This means the sugar is released more slowly. It's classed as an intrinsic sugar, not a free sugar like the biscuit, and is packed with vitamins and minerals.

So for the calories/sugar, you get a whole lot more with the apple than the biscuit. (And let's face it – it's so easy to eat more than one biscuit, which further increases your sugar and fat intake.)

Here's a little experiment. Choose two consecutive days where your activity is more or less the same. On the first day, eat an apple, ideally as a snack and not part of a meal. Make a note of how long it takes you to eat it and when you next feel hungry. How much time lapses between eating the apple and you feeling hungry again?

On the second day, do the same but with a chocolate biscuit (just one). Did you notice any differences in how long it took you to eat the two foods? And how long before you felt hungry following each? Was there a difference? I'm guessing the apple took longer to eat and kept you fuller for longer. Were you tempted to have more than one biscuit? I bet you didn't even contemplate having more than one apple.

Make friends with soluble fibre, which is what's in the apple – it keeps you fuller for longer, is great for your gut bacteria, keeps your bowels regular and stops you overeating. It's the dietitian's top-secret way to get people to eat less and feel fuller. *(Shhhh, don't tell anyone I told you!)*

People often say, 'Well, fruit has loads of sugar in

it.' And it's true. That's why it tastes sweet. But as I explained above, you get so much more for your sugar calories as long as you're eating the fruit in its whole state. We should be aiming for a minimum of five servings of fruit and veg a day. If you can get more in, great (up to 10). Whole fruit is a great snack three times a day, and veg can be packed into any sauce and hidden nicely.

FRUIT VS. SMOOTHIES VS. JUICE

In today's world of juicing and smoothie mania, we have started to process fruits and vegetables to make them more convenient to take. However, this has doubled or tripled the portions we're eating. And in the case of juicing, we're removing the pulp, which has all the lovely soluble fibre we talked about earlier. But surely it's good to be eating more fruit and veg?

The rule is whole fruit is better than smoothies or juices, as it's both harder to overeat and it's the least processed. However, if you're struggling to include fruit or veg in your diet, then smoothies are the next best way to increase your intake.

Only have small amounts at a time (150ml) so you're not overdoing the portions. And don't over process it and remove all the pulp (fibre).

In an ideal world, you'd have a mixture of whole fruit, smoothies and juices. A trick I play with smoothies is to get two or three types of veg in (like kale, spinach and carrot) and then add just 1 fruit, or even half a portion. That way you're maxing out the veg without going overboard on the fruit sugar.

COMPLEX CARBOHYDRATES

Simple sugars are the first type of carbohydrate. Complex carbs are the other..

Examples of complex carbs include rice, potatoes, pasta, cereals, pittas, naan bread, chapattis, wraps, tortillas and bread. These foods, particularly bread, have received such bad press. (Remember the trainer calling them 'the devil's food'?)

Why and how does your body use and need complex carbs? And how are they different to sugars? Why do we need carbs? We can get energy from fats and protein, so what's the difference? When I cut carbs out I lose weight, so they can't be good for us, can they?

These are all questions I get asked regularly. So let's answer them.

Complex carbs, or starchy foods as they're also termed, are the human body's primary source of energy. That means our bodies are designed to use this food as the best and main source of fuel. When we eat starchy foods, they travel down to our stomachs, which takes around 20 minutes (depending on what you're eating them with and the type, e.g. wholegrain or white).

The starchy food hits your stomach, which then digests it and breaks down the starch into sugars. Yes, complex carbs are made up of chains of sugar molecules that need to be broken down by stomach enzymes. They're a bit like a string of pearls, where the individual pearls are the sugar molecules and the threads holding the pearls together make the sugar into starchy foods. Hence, they don't taste sweet. The first difference between sugar and starch digestion is that starches take more effort, and therefore energy, to digest. (Remember – sugar digestion starts in the mouth, not the stomach.)

The sugar from the starch is then able to pass from the stomach to the blood. The scientific term is actually glucose when it's in the blood, hence the term 'blood glucose'. It's then carried around that motorway system to the different parts of the body, where it's needed for energy. All parts of our body, especially the brain, prefer to use sugar as their number one energy source. Signs of hunger – like lack of concentration, stomach pangs, dizziness, irritability (I even had a patient describe it as 'hangry') – are all signs of low blood glucose. It's your body's way of saying, 'The tank is empty, so please refuel.'

Do you regularly ignore those signals? Or even notice them? I often hear patients say, 'I'm too busy,' or 'I'm going out for a meal tonight and so I'm saving myself.' And then they complain of sugar cravings or eat everything in sight when they get home. That's like expecting your car to drive you to work and back on no fuel, and then you dumping too much fuel in when you get home. Crazy, right? Your car isn't going to get you very far, very efficiently.

Yet daily I hear people say they never eat breakfast or often skip lunch – and then complain of fatigue or lack of concentration. Then when they get home, their blood sugars are so low that their brain's screaming for a very quick fix. So what's the quickest way to get your blood sugar up? You guessed it! Simple sugars. Why?

Because they're absorbed from the mouth. That's why you grab the sweetest (and usually high fat) thing you can find – like chocolate, biscuits or cakes

– and eat it at a rate of knots. It's not your fault: your brain needs fuel and it needs it quickly. But you could have avoided all that if you had prevented your body and brain from getting to that point – by eating regularly.

You can avoid this cycle with regular intakes of starchy foods throughout the day, and you will probably eat fewer calories and less fat. A chocolate bar can be anywhere from 200 to 500 kcals depending on the size, compared to a slice of bread at around 100 kcals (never mind the sugar and fat differences). So, thinking you're being really healthy by not having that bread or that small serving of pasta with your lunch means that you're eating way more later in the day, when you're least likely to burn it off. Double whammy.

Then we have the carb-haters group who say, 'I've had my omelette for breakfast and my chicken/tuna/salmon salad for lunch. That's healthy, right?'

That's like running a petrol car with diesel. It's the wrong fuel. Your body might work for a while, but the signs of low blood sugar will start because you're not providing your body with the vital fuel (carbs) that it needs. The key to fuelling your body correctly is to have a portion of starchy food at each meal; ideally a quarter to a third of what's on your plate should be starch. This will prevent you from overeating later in the day, which will help keep your weight down and in a healthy range. It will also stop you from turning into an afternoon/night-time sugar monster.

And this is when I hear a massive: 'Oh my God, that makes perfect sense. That's what I've been doing! No wonder I'm not getting the results I want!'

In summary, don't avoid meals and don't avoid starchy foods at mealtimes. Your brain needs them to prevent you grabbing high-calorie, low-nutrient foods later.

CHAPTER TWELVE

PROTEIN, PROTEIN, PROTEIN

THE WONDER FOOD. THE KEY TO EVERY DIETER'S WEIGHT-LOSS DREAM.

But what is protein? What does it actually do? How much do we actually need?

Protein gives us vital amino acids, which build our muscles

Protein is a macronutrient, which means it's a nutrient we need daily and in large amounts, just like carbs and fat. Our muscles are made from amino acids. Humans need nine essential amino acids to survive, and these are found in protein-rich foods. In fact, protein-rich foods are the only places our bodies can get amino acids. So, it's really important you have a good source of protein at each meal. It's even more important for growing bodies, as not only do they need to repair the existing muscle but they're growing more muscle. Think teenagers, children and babies. Remember: if your teenagers are choosing fizzy drinks over meals, they're fuelling with poor quality energy and missing vital nutrients. You can't be an Arnold Schwarzenegger without those essential amino acids.

Surprisingly, we only need between 12 and 15% of our total energy from protein. About 0.8 to 1g per kilogram of body weight is the recommended daily allowance (RDA) for adults in the UK. So if you weigh 80 kg, then you need about 60 to 80g of protein a day. That actually isn't a great deal if you think that a chicken breast, lamb chop or large tin of baked beans is around 20g.

Also, a meal containing more than 30g of protein is pointless because the body can only use up to 30g at once. The surplus protein is broken down by the body and used as a secondary energy source, and those essential amino acids I talked about earlier are broken down into nitrates and passed into your urine. Basically, it's a waste of time and money eating a meal that has more than 30g of protein.[25]

PROTEIN WON'T WORK UNLESS YOU HAVE CARBS, TOO

Many people make the mistake of thinking a meal of mainly protein and veg with no carbs is really healthy. Think again. I have had many gym bunnies and guys come to me saying, 'I'm eating really healthily and have a really high-protein, low-carb diet, but I'm not building the muscle I want and I feel like I have no energy. I don't understand why, because I'm training regularly!'

Well, the reason is that protein needs energy for your body to make muscle. A meal high in protein with no carbs means your body is prioritising energy for essential functions like breathing and your heart beating over building muscle. It's feeding the brain and all your vital organs before building your washboard abs. Therefore, a meal that has no real fuel (carbs) means that all that lovely muscle-making protein is used for energy first, and the amino acids are peed out because fuel is more important than muscle making. So, that expensive steak or lamb chop would have been better as a potato or some pasta. It's about having the right combination on the plate so the carbs feed the brain and body and help the protein do its job of making and repairing muscle.

An ideal plate for the average adult would be ¼ carbs, ¼ protein (no more than 30g) and ½ veg or salad, as a rough guide. This will help you get the best from that muscle-building protein via three meals a day.

THE BEST TYPES OF PROTEIN

So now that we're using the protein for muscle building and repair and not energy, let's talk about the best types of protein to get those nine essential amino acids I talked about earlier.

Animal sources of protein like meat, poultry and fish all contain the essential amino acids and are thus classed as high-biological-value protein foods. Eggs actually have the closest combination of essential amino acids for humans, which is why a lot of body builders eat them.

'But I'm a vegetarian,' I hear you say. 'Am I doomed?'

No, although you need to put in a little more thought. All nine essential amino acids are found in plant-based foods but not in any single food with the exception of soya. So you need to eat a variety of plant-based sources, like pulses, seeds, nuts, dairy and eggs (if you eat them).

Get creative and experiment with different proteins

– remember, variety is the spice of life. That goes for meat eaters as well as veggies. The more varied the range of foods you eat, the more nutrients you get and the healthier you feel. It's recommended that we have at least one meat-free day a week for good health and to sustain the world's supply of animal-based protein. There is also loads of other health benefits for a more plant-based diet and less meat - from better pooping habits, to healthier heart, reduced cancers and healthier skin. I challenge you meat-heads to that. See if you can get the same amount of protein for at least 1 day a week by eating veggie sources. After all, it's great for you (getting you closer to your 10 a day) and great for the environment! Win/win, I say.

THE MYTH OF THE HIGH-PROTEIN, LOW-CARB DIET

I often get asked 'If I eat a high-protein, low-carb diet, I lose weight. How does that work then?'

Well, if you exclude any macronutrient (nutrients we need daily in large amounts), you will lose weight because you're missing out a whole food group. It would work the same if you missed out protein and only ate carbs. The difference is that proteins make your feel fuller for longer and increase your satiety hormones, so you don't tend to overeat. On the other hand, depending on the type of carbs you have, it's easier to overeat and become deficient in those nine amino acids.

Basically, eating loads of protein and veg is easier that eating a high-carb, low- protein diet. But it's hard to sustain because it tends to be lower in fibre, which means it can play havoc with your bowels and leave you craving refined high-sugar snacks like chocolate. Ring any bells?

The number of patients who think they're addicted to chocolate/sugar/sweets is unbelievable. Then I explain that their brain is being deprived of the right fuel – carbs – so it's just getting desperate and responding to low blood sugars, leading to sugar cravings. The minute they start having balanced meals, their cravings stop and they come back saying 'I'm cured! It's like magic!'

Also, it's important to note that complex carbs and protein have roughly the same number of calories per gram (not that I'm encouraging calorie counting, because I'm not). The only reason I mention this is to combat the misconception that protein is lower in calories than complex carbs. But they're the same. So if you load your plate with filling protein while your body desperately wants pasta or pizza, you may actually be eating more calories in protein than you think. And remember from the last chapter – because your body prefers carbs as its primary fuel, the sugar (simple carbs) you crave and eat later actually has four calories per gram and gives you no other nutrients.

I had a *Grace who was consuming what she thought was a really healthy diet – low carbs (so she thought), high protein and lots of veggies. She couldn't work out why she was so moody and was putting on weight. Generally, the only meal she loved was her breakfast, which was avocado, egg and seeded toast. She would find herself gorging in the evening and always needing a sugar fix at 3pm.

Can you identify with some of her issues? Do you think she was following a low- calorie diet?

She was actually overeating and having more calories in sugary foods because she was so hungry. Her body was craving carbs, and she would have been better off including a small amount of complex, good-quality carbs with each meal and reducing her protein intake slightly. Yes, I'm saying the meal she loved the most was balanced! Yes, I'm saying eat whole-wheat pasta, baked potatoes, seeded bread and the occasional pizza. They'll reduce your craving for the empty, crappy, nutrient- lacking sugary and fatty foods like chocolate, cakes and biscuits.

Now I'm not saying you shouldn't ever eat those treats. That's not the point of Food Freedom. I live in the real world – you don't think dietitians eat those foods? We love them like everyone else. The difference is that with Food Freedom they don't control you, they're not like a drug you're addicted to. When you eat them, you enjoy them and therefore only need a small amount.

Let me give you another example of *Joyce who couldn't stop eating four chocolate bars a day. Just think about how much sugar and fat that is daily. She hated the compelling feeling and the lack of control.

Within two weeks of balancing her meals, she couldn't remember when she last had a chocolate bar. It's not magic – just basic physiology. Put your body in the right state, fuel it correctly and the rest will follow.

EATING PROTEIN TO CHANGE YOUR BODY SHAPE

So what's the ideal amount of protein to sustain weight or shift your body composition to more lean tissue (muscle) and less fat?

The current evidence suggests that while 0.8g per

kilogram of body weight is the RDA, just slightly increasing your intake to 1.2 to 1.6g per kilogram makes you more likely to gain muscle and reduce fat, especially belly fat.[26] However, this depends on how active you are and what type of exercise you're doing – be it weight-bearing, cardio or a mixture. (That's a whole new book and not my area of expertise.)

DIMPLE'S FIVE
PROTEIN RULES

1. Combine protein with carbs to get the most benefit.

2. Vary the source of protein – so not always chicken for dinner.

3. Don't eat more than 30 g per meal – you only need roughly 1.2 to 1.6 g per kilogram of body weight a day, so don't be tempted to overdo it and compromise your complex carbs.

4. Be creative to ensure you get all 9 essential amino acids – this is especially important if you're vegetarian because your protein sources have fewer amino acids each.

5. Enjoy meals that are ¼ protein, ¼ carbs and ½ veg or salad as a general rule.

CHAPTER THIRTEEN

FATS: GOOD OR BAD?

As a dietitian, a question I get asked constantly is: 'Is butter good for you or not?' So let's get the story straight on fats. Fats fall into three categories: monounsaturated, saturated and polyunsaturated. Within polyunsaturated, there are two groups: omega 6 and omega 3.

All fats provide us with essential fatty acids, which are necessary to keep us fit and well. Vital organs like our heart and lungs have a layer of protective fat around them, kind of like a shock absorber. Our skin has a layer of fat underneath (some of us have a thicker layer than others), and this acts as an insulator and keeps us warm. Nerves are also covered in a tube of fat, a bit like the plastic casing found around electrical wires. This tubing acts in the same way as the plastic on the electrical wires – it stops the brain's electrical messages from escaping and helps the impulse reach the right part of the body. This could be the brain asking a muscle to move or the heart to beat.

So yes, we do need fats in our diet. But we're over-consuming fats massively for the following reasons:

1. Fats make food taste good because they can act as an Emulsifier, binder and flavour carrier

Over the decades, the food industry has used more of them in convenience products. As the amount of processed foods we eat has increased and we move away from cooking from scratch, we don't have as much control over how much fat is on our plates.

2. Diet fads are encouraging fat consumption

With the popularity of diets like the Atkins diet, people have been given permission to eat more fat from all three groups.

3. Food has become faster and more mobile

We're snacking more, especially on high-fat, high-sugar foods instead of eating sit-down meals. You will learn more in later chapters on why this means you eat more of everything, including fats.

This overeating of fats isn't good because they're the highest calorie nutrient.

FAT: kcals per Gram of fat

CARBS: 3.5 kcals per gram of fat

PROTIEN: 4 kcals per gram of fat

That means that if you have 10g of fat on your plate, you have more than double the calories compared to 10g of protein or 10g of carbs. Why is that so bad? Well, it wouldn't be if you were burning those calories. But because fats taste so good, they're really easy to overeat, meaning you store them and put on weight. And being overweight is the harmful thing, not the fats themselves. Being overweight and leading an unhealthy, sedentary lifestyle can put you at greater risk of heart disease, diabetes and some cancers. (But we know all that, right?)

Let me tell you about *Joan. She had been yo-yo dieting from around age 13. She was approaching her 50's, was an amazing cook and had put her Air Steward's life on hold while she raised her three children. She had every diet book under the sun, had tried most and was familiar with spending hours cooking meals and snacks. And she was very confused, having had mainly chefs as her nutrition knowledge reference.

Joan came to me saying, 'I'm eating all homemade, healthy foods and snacks but my weight seems to be going up and up. Why?' She had an active life going to the gym and walking the dog daily – it seemed like a textbook recipe for weight loss. So what was the issue?

Well, when I looked at her diet, she was making these golf-ball-sized nut and seed balls daily, sometimes twice daily. When I asked for the ingredients, it became apparent that the fat content was very high – each was giving her almost 500 kcals a day. That's approximately a third of her daily intake! And some days she was eating two of them! While the fats were healthy, they were adding too many additional calories, and that was the cause of the weight gain. Joan stopped the nut balls immediately and replaced them with a piece of fruit. She lost weight but, more importantly, finally loves her body and the food she eats thanks to the Food Freedom model.

The bonus to Joan's story relates to her daughters. They were starting to develop relationships with food similar to those their mother had been modelling. Within a few months of Joan implementing the

Food Freedom model, everyone had much healthier language, mind-sets and intakes. In fact, two years on, the family have a phrase they use in their house – they say, 'We've been Dimpled!'

The moral of Joan's story is: if you want to add healthy fats to your diet, you need to swap them for something else. If you just add them on, you'll gain weight. So if you want to increase your healthy fat intake in the morning, change the way you make your porridge – halve your quantity of oats and replace them with a handful of linseeds. If you simply add the seeds, you'll double the calories in your breakfast.

The key to fats: keep them to a minimum and eat from all the types. You should reduce the overall amount of fat to avoid excess calories you don't burn off. But you should also have a healthy balance of fats.

Don't overdo the saturated fats. Use low-fat cooking methods and fats that are high in monounsaturates, such as olive or rapeseed oils. Monounsaturated fats are said to have a positive effect on fat profiles in your body, whereas saturated and polyunsaturated fats have a neutral effect. Within the polyunsaturated group, there is evidence to suggest that omega 3 fatty acids have less of an inflammatory response than omega 6.[27] This is behind the recommendation that we eat more oily fish (twice a week), linseeds, flaxseeds and walnuts. Keep it simple – this group of foods can put extra weight on you because it's so energy dense and tasty.

To give you an idea, here's what I do with fats. I keep fried foods to a minimum but on occasion love chips. I include flaxseeds and linseeds in my daily diet, and I have a mix of nut-based and dairy milk. So I vary where my fats are coming from to get a great blend while still enjoying my food.

That sums up the basic science behind food. Now let's move on to the psychology – why we eat what we eat.

CHAPTER FOURTEEN

WHAT IS MINDFUL EATING?

Mindful eating is a way of eating that focuses on 'how' and 'why' we eat rather than 'what' we eat.[28]

It's defined by paying attention to an eating experience with all our senses (seeing, tasting, hearing, smelling, feeling) – witnessing, without judgment, the emotional and physical responses that take place before, during and after the experience.[29] It's often discussed under the umbrella term 'mindfulness', the practice of increased awareness of our actions and our senses as they relate to the task at hand.

F or example, mindful breathing involves paying attention to our breathing, noticing how we move and feel and the impact of this purposeful breathing on our bodies.

HOW DOES MINDFUL EATING HELP YOU IMPROVE YOUR DIET, HEALTH AND WELLBEING?

The purpose of mindful eating is to move your focus away from the food and other external influences like time, place and people to explore the eating experience.[30]

When you do this you will notice the following things happen:

1. You will remember that you have eaten, rather than that feeling of 'Did I have lunch? I can't remember, so I'll have a biscuit.' That's what I call 'mindless' eating. When you're so busy that you don't notice how much or even what you've eaten, you're more likely to overeat high-calorie snacks.

2. You will start to enjoy your food more, and often this leads to being satisfied much earlier in the meal (and hence eating less).

3. You will engage your senses, first to notice and second to act upon your hunger and fullness signals, meaning you're less likely to overeat.

4. You will eat more slowly because you're focusing on all your senses while eating. You will notice how it tastes, what it smells like, the feeling the food gives you, how it feels in your mouth and stomach. This results in you eating less.

Mindful eating means you're more likely to eat what your body needs when it needs fuel, and you're less likely to overeat and put on unnecessary weight. It helps you keep a healthy weight for life!

WHAT'S THE POINT OF MINDFUL EATING?

Recent studies show that mindfulness is extremely helpful in promoting better eating behaviours, and that it assists with weight regulation.[31]

One study showed that mindful eating methods significantly reduced stress and fasting blood sugar in overweight and obese women.[32] Another, larger review found that mindful practices helped improve depression, anxiety, stress and quality of life.

Another study – this time of 8,683 people – found that use of mindfulness showed significant improvement in the treatment of cancer, cardiovascular disease, chronic pain, chronic somatic disease, depression, anxiety disorders and other medical disorders alongside traditional treatment paths. There were even improvements in healthy adults and children, too.[33]

Although more research is needed in this area, the results are promising. Who wouldn't want to reduce their stress and anxiety levels? Who wouldn't want to improve recovery rates for chronic conditions? Who wouldn't want to have a better relationship with food and regulate their weight? It's a no brainer, right?

Follow the four steps on the next page, and you'll get more enjoyment out of your food. You'll notice the benefits, which will encourage you to continue to eat in this way until it becomes second nature.

Remember – respect the fuel (food) and the fuel will respect you.

HOW DO YOU EAT
MINDFULLY?

1. Notice your hunger and full signals
Act on them, don't ignore them. Eat when you're hungry and stop when you're full. Both are equally important to avoid binging later.[34]

2. Move away from screens when eating
Eating while using a tablet, phone or TV means your focus is on the screen, not on the food or on how your senses are responding to the food. Distracted eating results in overeating.

3. Eat slowly, at half your normal speed
So, if it normally takes you five minutes to eat a meal, see if you can slow it down to 10 minutes. The ideal time is 20 minutes, as it takes approximately that long for your brain to fire your full feelings and signals.

4. Ensure your meals are balanced. Have veg/salad, protein and carbs as discussed in previous chapters. Your body needs all three elements to stay healthy and fuel itself.

CHAPTER FIFTEEN

WHO HAS THE CONTROL?

Is it you? Or the food?

Are you constantly thinking about your next meal or snack while still eating your current meal? Are you drawn to food outlets, cake shops or the sweet shop?

When did this happen? When did we let food take over our head space? And why?

Stop, pause, breathe and just notice who has control. Understand and be aware of what's actually going on. Are you eating when you're hungry? Do you even know when you're hungry or what hunger feels like? Do you allow yourself to get hungry, or are you always eating for fear of a sudden food shortage?

These are all questions and situations people find

themselves in when they feel food has the control. They're often very rational, successful people in all aspects of their lives except this. For some, this has been the habit of a lifetime and stems from when their parents would say things like:

'Finish what's on your plate.'

Or

'You're not leaving the table until you have finished everything. There are starving children in the world!'

And you would say, 'But I'm full!' And your well-intentioned parent would say, 'We don't waste food – eat up.'

Sound familiar? Maybe you're now that doting parent who wants to keep your child well-nourished and environmentally conscious!

Young children are very good at eating to hunger and stopping when full. They're not governed by time, media, celebs or magazine images. They're not aware of when it's lunchtime or breakfast. They just know when their bodies need fuel (hunger), when they have adequate fuel (full) and then act accordingly. They self-regulate depending on their bodies' varying needs. For example, if they're having a growth spurt, you hear parents say 'I can't fill them – they're eating me out of house and home!' or you might hear, when they're not growing, 'I don't know how they're surviving on the next to nothing they've eaten.'

The point of this explanation is that as we get older our external influences – school, work, schedules and parents – override our natural ability to eat when we're hungry and stop eating when we're full. We lose the ability to read those signals, or we ignore them for so long that we're deaf to them even when they're screaming to be heard.

Why?

Because life doesn't allow us to respond to them.

How often have you skipped lunch because you're too busy at work? Or had no time for breakfast because you had to get out the door?

Then you wonder why you aren't as productive in the afternoon, why your concentration levels are poor, or why you suffer with headaches?

Hello! Your body is screaming, 'Feed me!' And then

you go for the nearest sweet thing to fuel your brain fast. You've been expecting your car to run without fuel and then, when you finally give in and it's desperate, you dump a whole load of rocket fuel in it. You shoot like a rocket for about 30 minutes and then plummet as the high- energy fuel is used up. It's the quintessential sugar rush and crash.

So what exactly is wrong with this? You're getting fuel, right? You're eating, after all. Well, yes, you're eating, but the fuel you're choosing often has very little nutrient value for those calories. You get very few other vitamins and minerals and often a lot of fat. For example, a bag of sweets can give you anywhere from 300 to 500 kcals depending on the size and type. That's all it gives you. A sandwich made with granary bread, salad and some lean meat gives you roughly the same calories plus loads of protein, carbs, fibre, vitamins and minerals. It will fill you up and fuel your brain, and hence your productivity, for longer. With the sandwich, you're getting more value and satisfaction for your calories. Does that make sense?

HOW TO GAIN CONTROL

1. Notice how you do hunger

Do you feel it in your stomach or your head? I personally feel it in my head. I notice that my concentration goes and I start making mistakes at the task in hand. My head goes into what I call my hunger fog, and I can't think straight. For others, it's in their stomach: they describe it as a rumble and pain.

Everyone's body has its unique way of letting you know you're hungry. What's your hunger sign? Think back to a time when you were peckish, in the middle of something and some feeling in your body broke your concentration. It might just be for a second before you went back to the task. Go back to that feeling and locate it. Where do you feel it? Stomach, head, all over, where? What does it look like? Does it have a colour? Sound? Shape? Temperature? Does it move or is it still? Is it heavy or light? If you were to name it, what name might it be? Don't over-think it, just go with whatever pops into your head.

Now we have identified your hunger signal, we can do something about it. The key here is to ACT on it. When you feel it (because now you know what you're feeling and it has a name), EAT. Refuel your body. But make sure it's the right fuel. So, if it's near a meal time then have your meal; if it's in between, have a piece of fruit.

2. Don't ignore your hunger signal

Ignoring hunger leads to subsequent overeating on high-calorie, low-nutrient-value foods. So don't do it. It's not worth it. You will only increase your total calories for that day, turning to foods that lead to weight gain when you're not burning those calories off.

CHAPTER SIXTEEN

THINK LIKE A THIN PERSON

I n this chapter, we're going to talk about using neurolinguistic programming (NLP) as part of your diet.

NLP is a way of tapping into the resources you have within you but are unaware of. It's a vehicle that helps you amplify your skills and beliefs and helps you reach your goals. It's a bit like when you first learn to drive. You know the names of all the car parts (gear stick, clutch, etc.), but until you learn to use each part together your car won't move correctly. An NLP practitioner is like a driving instructor.

You can also use NLP when you're unsure of the goals you want to achieve or confused about which path to take to reach your objectives. It allows you to explore in a way you've never explored before, and take a road you never knew existed.

Think of it like a SATNAV and signs on the motorway once you've learned to drive. They help you decide where to go and how to get there.

One of the fundamentals of NLP, unlike other therapies, is that it embraces everything about you, even the aspects of yourself that frustrate you. Like the comfort-eating side of you, for example. It allows you to accept every part of you and helps you explain the good intention of that part – how it's helping and serving you. Once you accept every part of you and fully understand its purpose as part of your true self, the associated fight, emotions, guilt and frustration disappear. That part of you is now your friend, not your enemy.

Let's look at this in the context of food. There's that battle with wanting foods you know are 'bad' for you and you 'shouldn't have.' When you eat them, you tend to overeat – because you've started so you may as well finish. And then the guilt sets in. What if you accept that those so-called 'bad' foods are a healthy part of your diet - when they're in moderation and they serve a purpose, like as part of a birthday or a treat. Then you're more likely to enjoy less of them, and you won't feel the guilt. It won't affect your weight in the same way, so it helps you avoid sabotaging your success.

Here's an example of how I used NLP to help
*Mary deal with her constant battle with sabotage.
She knew her behaviour was preventing her from
achieving her goal but couldn't control the 'sabotage'
(as she referred to it). So we explored the function of
sabotage, its positive purpose for her. It turned out
it gave her pleasure. It was telling her to enjoy what
she was eating instead of wolfing down those 'bad'
foods so fast and in such large quantities that she
didn't even realise she had eaten them. All she was
experiencing was guilt and no pleasure! So sabotage
kept knocking at her door because she was totally
ignoring its purpose – to give pleasure when eating
the lovely foods she should be enjoying.

Have you ever decided to go somewhere but aren't
sure why? And then once you got there, it wasn't how
you imagined it would be? Or you set off on a journey
but obstacles just seem stop you from getting there?

This often happens when you set goals without
exploring their full impact. NLP helps you explore
your positive goals – like wanting to lose weight
or maintaining weight loss – in a new way. The
model uses well-informed outcomes to enable you
to experience how your goal will look, feel, sound
and smell to you and your significant others. So
when you're going for your goal, you know what it

will be like when you get there. You know how you will feel and how it will affect those around you. Often, this process shows people that their actual goal isn't weight loss but control over eating or a healthier relationship with food. Once the true goal is established and the end point looks, feels and sounds good, getting there becomes a piece of cake. (Excuse the pun, but everything in moderation – even cake!)

Often, as a result of identifying your real goal, weight loss or healthy weight maintenance becomes a by-product.

HOW DOES NLP WORK?

NLP is a series of models that help you explore areas in your life that you would like to change forever. It works on the principle that we develop neurological pathways to manage certain situations. These are learned and repeated over time, for example emotional eating when sad. NLP helps you rewire your learned natural responses to these situations.

So you might start by exploring other ways of managing that situation, then try out a few and decide on a new way of dealing with emotional eating. You do that until it becomes your normal pattern, and emotional eating is no longer a problem.

As your new pattern becomes part of your instinctive behaviour, values and beliefs, you then rewire to form a new learned neurological pathway and a new YOU.

I sometimes refer to it as 'thinking like a thin (or healthy) person.' It's a bit like when you first switch from full-fat milk to semi-skimmed milk. It tastes too watery at first, but then you get used to it. After a while, if somebody offers you full-fat milk, it tastes too fatty. Your taste buds have been rewired to prefer semi-skimmed.

INTRODUCING THE HUNGER SCALE

Ask yourself the following questions:

- Do you eat when it's time to eat even though you're not hungry?
- Do you often find yourself feeling bloated after meals?
- Do you always finish what's on your plate even if you're full?
- Do you find you've inhaled a meal so that you've not even tasted it or can't say what it was you ate?

Then the Hunger Scale Model is a fabulous tool for you.

The idea is that you learn how you do hunger and full. As we discussed in Chapter 15, we all have our own neurological signals for how we do hunger and full. NLP helps you to identify your own unique signs. Once you're familiar with your signals, you can use them to work with the Hunger Scale. *Source: Paul McKenna*[35]

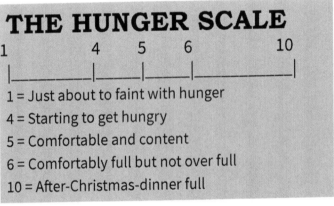

The Hunger Scale will challenge your beliefs, but the idea is that you form new beliefs and relationships with food to help you maintain a healthy weight for life. Once you get into this way for eating, you start to reap the benefits of clearer thinking, less fatigue, more energy, better sleep, regular bowel movements, less bloating and a healthier body size. And you're happier because you, not the food, have control of your eating.

I recently worked with a very successful young

businesswoman, *Sophia, who initially came to me saying she wanted a supermodel beach body (don't we all, lol – not!).

Once we delved deeper, it emerged that what she really wanted was to be less angry so she'd stop snapping at her staff. She had an amazing husband, but they were always focused on the next thing – they were never in the moment together.

We looked at her diet and soon realised that she spent most of her time between #1 and #4 on the Hunger Scale. This was when her blood sugar was low and dropping fast. She often ignored her #4 and pushed through, skipping lunch until 3pm, 4pm or even 5pm! Following some discussion on physiology and basic nutrition, she soon saw that there was a direct correlation between her mood and where she was on the Hunger Scale. The lower she was, the angrier (or should I say 'hangrier') she got.

So we developed a meal plan together, and she implemented it. Within a week, her goal of being less angry and more present was achieved. The power of the Hunger Scale is extraordinary. In my experience, allowing yourself to fall below #4 or go above #6 inevitably leads to overeating and unnecessary calories (whether or not they're healthy), which results in weight gain.

THE **HUNGER**
SCALE RULES

1. Only eat when you're at #4, which is when you experience your hunger signal – no matter what time it is.

2. Always stop when you're at #6, which is when you experience your full signal, even if there's still food on your plate.

4. Plan ahead to allow yourself to eat in this way – for example by having healthy snacks to hand.

6. Choose healthy foods 80% of the time, working on the 80:20 rule.

8. Eat slowly so you don't override your full signal with fast eating.

10. Notice and pay attention to your food – no screens at the table!

12. If you're unsure whether you're at #4 or #6, then stop eating. If you were at #4, the signal would be too strong to ignore. Chances are you're at #6. You can always eat again later if you feel your hunger signal again. The advantage to living in an affluent society is that food is always available!

THE 80:20 RULE

Old habits die hard, and we occasionally fall off the wagon and slip back into our old ways.

This is where the 80:20 rule comes in. This is when 80% of the time you're following the principles of Food Freedom and 20% of the time you aren't, for many reasons. For example, there's no veg or salad available where you are, you're at a party, it's a special occasion or you decide to have a day off. All these things happen, even to dietitians. It's called life.

The important thing is that you actually need to get back on the 80% - back on track. Here's why. When you're on the 20% it feels great – but with the up there is always a down. The return of the bloating, sluggish, uncomfortable, 'food hangover' feeling.

The hangover helps you get back on track and back to Food Freedom, a bit like an alcohol hangover stops you from drinking like that daily. Make sense? You need the 20% for 2 reasons:

1. To give yourself permission to have a life and flexibility, otherwise you would never go anywhere or do anything.

2. To have the food hangover to get you back on track – back on Food Freedom.

Following the 80:20 rule is a bit like first learning to drive a manual transmission car. You stall a lot, and it feels like it takes forever to restart the car. You have to put the handbrake on, take the car out of gear, turn the engine off and so on. It takes a few minutes but it feels like longer. Similarly, with the 80:20 rule, you have to reset your mind, take a breath, face your fears and frustrations and start the whole process again – knowing you will stall again. Soon you become so familiar with it that the stalling becomes less frequent, the recovery becomes quicker and the damage to your mind and wellbeing becomes less significant.

The more you practice Food Freedom, the less frequent the 20's become and the less time it takes for you to recover from them. So a 'bad' or 'naughty' day with eating (I never use these terms around food, by the way, because food is a necessity, not a luxury item) becomes less frequent, shorter lived and less damaging.

Instead of it taking you days to recover from a birthday or emotional eating episode, you just eat less than normal and don't allow it to sabotage the rest of your day. The 'Sod it, I've done it anyway so I may as well carry on' mind-set is replaced with, 'Oh well, I enjoyed that for what it was and now I'm back on track.' This results in fewer calories consumed and less time overeating.

I have a great example of this. I was doing a review with *Jane, and she told me her disabled daughter was in hospital again (unfortunately, a regular occurrence). She explained how her mind-set towards eating had been going out the window –Jane was piling on the weight she had lost and gaining more during these hospital stays. It was the equivalent to a massive stall that lasted days or even weeks.

However, during this hospital stay, she realised she had developed strategies using the Hunger Scale and the 80:20 rule – they gave her a fundamental structure to manage the situation. She accepted she was going to have days where she wasn't able to eat when she needed to and would maybe overeat later. By being aware of this, she was able to plan what she would eat and not mindlessly drive to the petrol station and have four chocolate bars!

Instead, she was in control. She had accepted the 80:20 rule and knew that a one-off, less-than-ideal meal or snack wouldn't have a massive impact. It would only affect her if she allowed it to continue for the full duration of the hospital stay and then for days after.

During this particular episode, she didn't gain any weight and was straight back to her Food Freedom plan and gym classes following her daughter's discharge. I would argue she never left the Food Freedom plan. Once on it, on it for life!

So, that's the 80:20 rule explained. Sometimes the 20% is for happy reasons like birthdays, but sometimes it's because we're emotionally uncomfortable, sad, bored, lonely, feel something is missing or just unaware.

The next chapter talks about emotional eating and a discovery I made while working with an amazing lady. Enjoy it (it's a good one)!

CHAPTER SEVENTEEN

FEED YOUR SOUL...
...NOT YOUR BELLY

OMG this is huge!

I discovered this phenomenon while working with my female patients. Many of them had grasped the concept of intuitive eating (eating to appetite) but still found themselves unhappy and doing emotional eating despite knowing they were full. What was going on? I needed to understand and explore more.

I was working with a stay-at-home mum, *Sue, who had a profoundly disabled child. She had come to me because she had lost herself in all the chaos of life as a carer. Impossible job, right? I mean, who can do that 24/7 and not serve themselves at any point? Her daughter was 8 years old, so she had done this for

8 years solid. Sue's husband worked and then every evening went to the gym, filled his soul and came home. She spent all day and night caring for her daughter and 12-year old son, and when the daughter was sleeping and the husband was at the gym she would eat.

Sue was lost in despair and trapped in a body that didn't belong to her.

After a few sessions, it hit me like a bolt of lightning. It was so clear. She was feeding her belly, not her soul. She had become so lost in the identity of being a loving mother, wife and carer that she had lost who she was! Her soul needed to be heard. She needed to serve it but instead was filling it with food. Quite literally pushing it back down into her belly with food. Does this sound familiar?

It happens when you comfort eat. The food may give comfort in the short term, but in the long term it sets off a whole cycle of feed, binge, discomfort and guilt. The feeling of unease is your soul calling. As it was for this lady.

As soon as we explored what was going on, she broke down with relief. Floods of tears – because for years she hadn't understood the why to the eating. The key to her behaviour had been unlocked. Sue was feeding her belly, not her soul.

So what came after the enlightenment? Did she wait for the universe to give her a sign of what to do next or how to sort out her situation? **NO.**

ACTION, ACTION, ACTION was needed.

We explored what it was her soul was calling for. She simply paused, asked and waited for whatever came.

For her, it was beautiful. She was a creative, witty soul with an amazing sense of humour. Her soul was calling her to lose herself in creating. Her things were sewing and reading. She had a sewing room in her house but never made or prioritised the time to sew and read, her greatest passions. When she talked about these (and they came to her straight away, by the way), she lit up. Her whole face, body and soul shone. She instantly sat up and giggled like a school girl who found she could sing like an angel and got the solo in the choir. She had discovered her love and had been given permission to practise it daily.

So, her homework for that week was to sew and read daily. We discussed in great detail how and when she would fit this in, basically replacing her binge time with soul time.

The following session was two weeks later. She had lost weight as a by-product of being happy. Her true self was emerging. She talked of her passion for what she had created. During her soul time, time stopped and flowed all at once. She was lost in her world of fulfilment, of sheer luxury. She said it was like eating cake but without the calories and guilt. Having your cake and eating it, I would say! While talking to her, I notice her face glowed. Her soul was free, no longer drowning in food and fat.

Shortly after the Christmas holidays, she returned. As soon as she walked through the door, I could tell she had lost her soul to food again. She sat slumped in the chair and just cried. She'd had a taste of a daily escape to paradise (only half an hour twice a day) and it had gone. Her weight had increased, and she was lost in a black cloud.

It soon became apparent that with the school holidays, her family were home and she had not communicated her need to feed her soul. She had not explained that when she went into her office/sewing room that it was her work, her time out. And so the family were paralysed without her – they needed their captain and the captain had not explained this shift. Her husband, David, had never managed the children alone and had no understanding of what needed to be done. She gave in to her family and old habits and started to feed her belly rather than her soul again. When you have had a taste of paradise and it's taken away from you, it's a harder pill to swallow. She burst into tears and said, 'All I want is to read my book in peace for half an hour!'

Her soul was calling. She needed to do the next step – prepare the troops and explain how she needed to feed her soul. She needed a team meeting where the captain could explain the shift in pattern and then go off for 30 minutes twice a day, handing over to her co-captain, her husband David.

Sue came back several weeks later. When we discussed soul work and whether it was still happening daily and consistently, she said, 'Of course it does, it's the law!' She even added that when she announced, the other day, that she was going to her sewing room, her son didn't even look up from his game and said, 'Do you need anything, David?' The child had become so used to mummy disappearing that he expected and conditioned the question she always asked! Soul work complete; permission granted from all those who mattered.

HERE ARE THE LESSONS:

THE TEN STEPS TO SERVING OUR SOUL
(SOS)

1. Recognise when you're feeding your belly instead of your soul.

2. Stop, pause and breathe.

3. Ask what your soul really, I mean really, needs.

4. Work out how, when and where.

5. Engage your troops and explain the shift

6. Go do it.

7. Form a new, non-negotiable ritual that you commit to daily, consistently and forever.

8. Make it so it becomes you. It's part of who you are. Your identity. Your soul. Your purpose.

9. Be YOU

10. Your physical being will emerge as the true you.

How do you know if you're feeding your soul and not your belly?

Feeding your soul feels good and feeding your belly when it's not hungry (remember your hunger signals) doesn't.

Don't be disheartened, because getting it wrong is just as important as getting it right. All feedback, especially negative, is an opportunity to change, grow, develop and move closer to your goal.

If you didn't have uncomfortable feedback like feelings of guilt and disappointment, then how would you know to change your behaviour? You have to feel uncomfortable in order to do something different. Does that make sense? You see, when you overeat, your body is telling you to stop and rethink what you're doing. The stop signal has to feel uncomfortable in order for you to pay attention. If it were comfortable and nice, you wouldn't stop.

Uncomfortable or negative feedback is your guide

to steer you back on course. Being back on course might be to notice what you're doing first, or might be to change your behaviour. Remember this equation from Chapter 3:

EVENT + RESPONSE = OUTCOME

The event may be out of your control, but you have control over your response and hence can influence the outcome. So if you always do what you always do, then you will always get the same outcome. If you choose to change your response to a situation, then you will get a different outcome.

The next time you notice you're moving towards filling your belly rather than your soul, stop, try to change your response and then take note of the outcome. You might just surprise yourself. You might just have a preferred outcome that serves your soul, not your belly!

CHAPTER EIGHTEEN

PRACTICE MAKES PERFECT

'Your brain sees no difference whatsoever between visualising something and actually doing it.'
Jack Canfield, author of The Success Principles

WHAT IS VISUALISATION AND WHAT'S THE POINT?

Visualisation is when you play the story/outcome you want in your head. You notice the good stuff and live as if you have it already.

This technique has been used for many years to train Olympic athletes; they imagine they've run the race as if they've won. A lot of successful people use it. You hear them say, 'I just "see it,"' or 'I just know it's going to happen.' How do they know? In their mind's eye, it's already happened – and they know how to make it happen.

HOW DOES VISUALISATION WORK?

'How can this possibly work?' I hear you say. 'How can I think myself thin?' Visualisation is a well-documented tool that psychologists use, and it works on the following model.

VISUALISATION

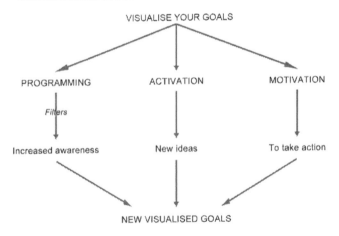

Let me explain how it works. You visualise something, which alters the programming in your brain, which in turn adjusts your filters. Filters are what we use every day to organise the thousands of messages that bombard us. Our brain uses a system of filters that allows us to make sense of all these messages and prioritise, delete and organise as relevant to us.

Do you remember when you decided to do something for the first time – buy a new car, think about having a baby, look for a new house – and suddenly you started noticing the car you wanted or pregnant ladies or every single for-sale sign?

Weird, right? How suddenly all these things magically appeared! Well, they haven't magically appeared – they've always been there. Your filters have altered because your programming is different. And it's because your visualisation has changed to imagining yourself in the new car or holding that baby or enjoying your new house. Your filters have changed to reflect your new goals, which has increased your awareness of what you want. This makes you more likely to achieve that visualised goal in reality.

The second thing that happens when you visualise your goal is that your brain starts to activate new ideas. For example, you start to think about ways you can get the new car, how you would adapt your life to a baby, what route you would take home from a new house. All these thoughts are activated by your new visualisation and your filters, allowing you to see things that were already there.

The third thing that happens is you're super motivated to achieve the goal, so you take decisive action to get there. You start thinking about how you're going to pay for the car and you visit showrooms or look at cars on the Internet. Suddenly you start noticing other pregnant ladies and chatting to them or reading blogs about being a new mum. Or you start researching the area that you'd like to live in and discussing mortgages. You can see how visualisation compels you to think about your goal, giving you ideas on how you to get it and motivating you to act.

Now I'd like you to think about the time you achieved the biggest goal in your life. This could be as a child acing your spelling tests or passing your exams. Or it could be as an adult getting your first job.

Take a moment to reflect on the process you used to get your goal. Was there a moment when you visualised it? Did you suddenly start noticing others around you who have already achieved it? Did this inspire you to have new thoughts and ideas on how you might take the next step? And then, did this motivate you?

This very same principle works when it comes to achieving the body and the relationship with food you long to have.

By constantly visualising yourself as 'the big boned girl' who's 'always been fat,' you're prompting your brain to set filters. So you only see the cake shop, the heavier girls or images of yourself a bigger size than you want to be. You never see the images of you actually being the size that's true to you. All your ideas are focused on losing weight and how you can restrict yourself. Your motivation to take action is then aimed at maintaining, if not gaining. And you remain the same size/weight as your visualisation. So, you're almost using visualisation in reverse by allowing it to stop you from achieving your true goal.

Visualisation can be a breakthrough moment for my patients because they've never truly visualised themselves as their true size or weight. When we do the exercise, they see for the first time who they're actually meant to be, their true authentic self. It's a tearful and emotional moment (for both of us, usually).

Visualisation will only take 10 to 15 minutes of your day. You get the maximum benefit if you can do it straight after meditating.

EIGHT **STEPS** TO
VISUALISATION

1. Know your goal.

2. Close your eyes and visualise it.

3. Add colour, sound, movement,
   smell and taste

4. Really feel it. How does this environment make
   you feel? How do the clothes feel on your back,
   against your waist? And how does that make
   you feel?

5. Bask in the feelings and revel in the full-colour
   images. This is the most important part.

6. If you're struggling to visualise, print some
   images or symbols of your vision – like a dress
   you want to wear or clothes you'd love to fit
   into again once you're the size you want to be.

7. Repeat, repeat, repeat 2 - 3 times a day.

8. Put the images somewhere you'll see them
   daily, like on the fridge, desk or bedside table.

THE FOOD FREEDOM QUADRANT

The Food Freedom Quadrant shows the direct correlation between Food Freedom, food noise and weight change. This isn't a scientific cycle – it's an anecdotal quadrant I developed to help my patients understand the relationship between all the components of Food Freedom and control. Here's how it works:

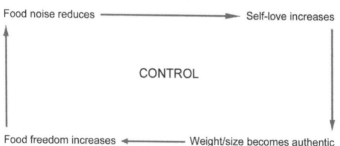

I codified the Food Freedom Quadrant for patients who were concerned about falling off the food-freedom wagon.

Let me give you an example. *Elizabeth had been on the programme for six months and recently noticed her weight creeping up and food noise increasing.

She also noticed she was feeling out of control and was starting to slip back into her old dietary habits of listening to media nutrition messages, missing meals and being tempted with detox diets. Her mind was becoming confused by the weight gain. She was emotional and upset, and I could see she was describing feeling unaligned. She was experiencing the reverse of Food Freedom It was the exact opposite of where she wanted to be on the Food Freedom Quadrant.

We talked through the Food Freedom Quadrant and what had happened. Understanding the relationship between all the components made her realise that to regain control she simply needed to pick up her tools and follow the quadrant in a clockwise direction. She needed to remember her #4 and #6 Hunger Scale triggers, trust them and action them. She needed to remember her sabotage messages, recall her soul animal, daily rituals, reasons for maintaining the animal and refocus. It was as clear as crystal to her.

Because she understood the elements of the Food Freedom Quadrant and how they were related, she had the tools to get back on the programme.

In fact, she always had the tools, she had just forgotten to use them. Within a week, she was back to the size she was happy with and, most importantly, felt in control. Her sense of Food Freedom had returned. The direction of flow had switched from anticlockwise to clockwise. Harmony was restored.

CHAPTER TWENTY

WHAT OTHERS NOTICE WHEN YOU HAVE FOOD FREEDOM

You're probably wondering why this chapter is in here and what it has to do with how you choose to eat, drink and relate to food and your body. Well, most of us live in a family or social network. As human beings, we surround ourselves with significant others who impact our lives – and believe it or not, we impact on theirs.

WE NEED TO TALK ABOUT FEEDBACK

How do you respond to feedback? I mean good and bad feedback? Have you ever noticed? Like when somebody says, 'Oh, are you on your next diet?' or 'You've tried to lose weight before – what makes you think this will work?'

Does this leave you feeling angry? Sad? Do you just ignore them? Or do you take it on board and action it?

Feedback is just somebody letting you know their opinion. You decide how and what you do with it (remember the equation: Event + Response = Outcome). You can choose to be angry or sad, but does that help you stay on track? Or does it make you emotionally eat or alienate the person giving the feedback? How you choose to process feedback may influence your ability to stay focused on your goal of Food Freedom.

Jack Canfield[36] suggests we see feedback as an opportunity to get honest insight into our behaviour from someone who's brave enough and loves us enough to express it to us. I'm not talking about unhelpful feedback (although even that can be useful).

For example, when your mother says, 'You're always on a diet, and they just don't work for you.' You could take that as, 'She has no faith in me and thinks I'm fat.' Or, 'What does she know?' Or, 'It upsets me when my mum judges me and thinks I'm fat.' Or, you could decide to think:

'Thank you, mum, for your observation. You're right that I've had a lifetime of diets that have made me feel bad and supported my weight gain. So today I choose to do something different. Something that makes me feel good and I know will take care of my weight so it reaches where it should be. Thank you so much for reminding me that diets don't work for me.'

BY CHOOSING TO TAKE THE FEEDBACK IN A CONSTRUCTIVE WAY, THREE THINGS HAPPEN

1. You're grateful to, not angry at, the person giving you the feedback, so you don't push them away (this is important, as often they're a loved one).

2. You're in a better state to remain focused on your goal because you're armed with new information and knowledge.

3. You have new insight into your behaviours and can choose how to manage that information to help you reach your goal of Food Freedom.

THE 5 GROUPS OF PEOPLE THAT WILL NOTICE YOUR FOOD FREEDOM...

Now let's look at what people may start to notice when you have Food Freedom. I've split this into 5 groups, but there's overlap. This is just meant to give you possibilities that may result from your new relationship with food.

1. Your partner/spouse/significant other

This usually falls into two camps: the supportive and encouraging one and the 'What's going on? Everything is changing and I don't think I like it' one.

Let's start with the positive supporter. You'll hear things like: 'I've never seen you so happy and focused and well.' 'You're glowing!'

'You look so healthy and happy.'

'You seem much calmer and happier when we're eating.' 'Life is so much easier now around food.'

'Remember when we couldn't eat at this restaurant because nothing was on your diet?'

This is all feedback, and you get to decide how you take it. My interpretation is:

Your spouse has noticed a shift in your behaviour

towards food because of your shift in beliefs. They've noticed the absence of all your unhealthy, self-limiting behaviours around food – those things that stopped you from living your life, going to the restaurants you wanted and eating the foods you love (like bread!). They're giving you feedback on the impact of truly feeding your body though intuitive eating, that it's had an impact on your behaviour, state and therefore relationship with your spouse. This is all positive. You should embrace it and see it as a step in the right direction to serving your true self. It's also a reason never to go back to food noise and a reason to keep Food Freedom.

Now for the second type of feedback you might get from a spouse: 'Why aren't you eating all that?'

'I can't believe you aren't having a dessert.' 'Why don't you want supper?'

'We always have supper! What do you mean you aren't hungry?' 'What do you mean you're having some time to yourself?'

'Why have you stopped drinking? Why are you having water?'

In this situation, the shift in your beliefs and behaviour around food has left your partner lost. Some even liken it to a bereavement. They've lost their 'eating and/or drinking buddy.' They're essentially saying, 'Whoa! What's going on? We had this wonderful relationship with food together and now you don't want to play. Why? I don't understand.'

Your partner may be feeling lost and redundant, so the feedback may present in a negative way. Remember that it's feedback, and you're the one who decides how you respond and react. You can choose to take it personally and get upset. At best, this will leave you stuck in an unhelpful state. At worst, this will make you feel bad and perhaps deflated about your progress, which could result in a relapse where you slip back into old, unhelpful behaviours. (NOOOO! All that hard work!)

You must start by being aware that you have a choice, that your partner is just giving you feedback and that it's not personal – they're just expressing their concerns because things have changed. Then you can move your relationship and your partner's relationship with food forwards to a much healthier one. I call this the ripple effect. Food Freedom has no barriers and can therefore impact anyone and everyone.

If you're in this position with your spouse, I suggest trying the following:

1. Turn off the angry button because two angry

people just create an avalanche.

2. Pause and think, 'What's my end goal? Is it to fight and be right, or is it to be happy and have loving relationships with my partner, food and my body?'

3. Notice that your behaviour has changed for the better, moving towards your goal of Food Freedom.

4. Acknowledge the feedback and thank your partner for it. Discuss the part that has had an impact on the dynamics of your relationship.

5. Explain the Food Freedom model and why under-eating and overeating are no longer options for you. It might be worth explaining intuitive eating and how it works. You never know – they may start mimicking you to address their own food noise.

6. Explain why this way of eating is now the norm for you. Describe all the benefits, like a healthier body, feeling in control, reduced emotional eating and less bloating and discomfort.

7. Explain that your feelings for them have not changed and that you're still the same person. You still want to share food but in a different, more aligned way. Maybe you also want to explore different non-food activities together. I've had couples decide to take up walking again or learn how to cook new healthier foods, for example.

8. It's important they hear and feel that you still love them. That you want to share this experience with them and would be very grateful for their support.

9. Make them feel included and part of the journey. It gives them a role in the new dynamic.

10. Check in with them from time to time. Ask how they feel about the situation. Is there anything that could improve?

11. Start to enjoy the journey of learning and discovery together. Often the Food Freedom message is transferred to your loved ones. What a gift – the gift of food love.

2. The feeder in the family (could be your mother/ father/sister/brother)

You may be hearing things like:

'I've brought you some leftover cake I couldn't finish it and know you'll eat it.'

'I couldn't resist the buy-one-get-one-free offer on these chocolates, so I bought you one as I can't possibly eat both.'

'I've booked us in to that favourite all-you-can-eat buffet. We can have a cheat day!'

You may find yourself constantly having to side-step

these gestures of goodwill and love. You may find yourself getting upset, annoyed or frustrated at your caring relative.

WHAT'S HAPPENING HERE AND HOW DO YOU RESOLVE IT?

As with the partner, there's a shift in roles in the relationship. The feeder may be showering you with love through food. It may be the way they've always shown their affection and now you're rejecting it. (Well, not really – but it may seem like that in their eyes.)

You're doing something different and they're doing what they've always done. It's a bit like when you transition from primary school to high school. At first your mother needs to walk you to school and hold your hand. Then the day comes when you don't want her to hold your hand because you're a big girl. Eventually you don't even need her to walk you. It's a transition of roles, and feelings of anger, frustration, rejection and confusion can arise when this happens. It's called growth.

The same thing happens when you have Food Freedom – you don't need to hold hands anymore. You've graduated high school. You're no longer dependant on a feeder to show you love through food. Just remember that the feeder has had years of giving love this way, and so adjusting to your new-found behaviour (in a relatively short space of time) may leave them feeling redundant. So be mindful of that.

Explain that you no longer need the extra food and that you can develop new ways of sharing love and time. Imagine the options and the money saved on the buy-one- get-one-free offers! Explain your Food Freedom and what it means to you. Use the 10- step guide in the partner section above – it works just as well here. Understand what your loved one's needs are – is it showing love? Is it displacing calories from themselves? Share the Food Freedom message. You never know: they might just decide to follow suit!

I had a lady called *Jaz whose mother would always bring cakes and biscuits round because she had bought them and didn't want to eat them herself. She was unintentionally sabotaging her daughter's progress with love. At first Jaz didn't want to hurt her mother's feelings, so she would just accept the gifts and either eat them or give them to her children. Jaz soon realised that she had to face her mother in a kind but firm way. She was assertive and simply asked her mother to take the goodies home and stop buying them. No one was eating them, she said, it was a waste of money. A better gift would be a day out with the children. That was the end of the sabotaging behaviour and the start of some amazing memories.

3. Well-meaning friends and colleagues

This is the friend who's been your diet buddy for years and is on the latest fad diet, is losing half her body weight a week and is explaining to you how easy it is. If you just spend half your monthly salary on all these wonderful pills, potions, shakes and products and stop eating real food for a week you, too, will lose the weight! You hear her getting compliments and you're tempted to follow suit because Food Freedom doesn't focus on rapid weight loss (and wasn't that why you went for Food Freedom?).

No. Stay focused on why you started the Food Freedom process. It was to gain control of your eating and have a healthier relationship with food forever. **NOT** to focus on losing weight fast. Because now you know that 'diets' just make you fatter in the long run!

I suggest you just wait and see what your friend's weight is in six months. Is she happy, doing the things she wants and still maintaining the size she wants to be?

You can choose to keep the feedback she's giving you at arm's length or you can internalise it. Find something new to share with your friend. Or find new friends whose common ground with you isn't dieting. Life moves in different cycles, and if you surround yourself with people you want to be like, then you're more likely to succeed in your goals. Move on if you need to, or share the Food Freedom love. You're in control of your response to the feedback.

> ### *Be grateful for the bad stuff because it gives you the opportunity to choose the stuff that feels right for YOU*

4. Media madness

Have you always been tempted or seduced by the latest celeb diet? Or the latest juicing product? Or an ad on social media claiming the magic tea will help you lose half your body weight in a week? (It's a slight exaggeration, but you know what I mean.)

Well these are all tests of your ability to enforce your new-found Food Freedom mind- set. They're testing your knowledge, beliefs and ability to know what's right for you.

Let me tell you about *Joan. This lady was highly successful and driven in her career, and made a massive difference to many lives. She had yo-yo dieted for 30 years, spending approximately £50,000 and remained a size 20 to 22. Joan was going from one diet to the next, losing and putting on weight, but never really gaining control or getting the food noise to a comfortable level. She was unaware of how destructive food noise and dieting were for her – she was constantly fighting with her true self, and this was manifesting itself in feeding her belly and not her soul. Not a great place to be.

Her mind-set around dieting and weight management/loss had always been: 'It has to be hard for it to work.'

'Dieting isn't easy.'

'If you're on a diet then you can't eat and do the things you love.' 'You need special foods that cost a lot of money to lose weight.' 'I will always be trying to lose weight.'

'If that diet worked for my friend, it will work for me.'

Following three sessions with me, she shifted her mind-set to Food Freedom. Her food noise reduced from 100% to 20%, a healthy, controllable amount.

And it was positive food noise around intuitive bodily cues rather than external cues. Joan started losing weight steadily while still enjoying Christmas, holidays, weekends away and meals out. She couldn't believe she had become that person – the one who says no to dessert because they're full or leaves half of her meal.

She felt in control, but in the back of her mind she had some doubts: 'This won't last. It's too good to be true. Why aren't I losing weight faster, like on all the other diets?'

Joan began to lose sight of her progress because of all those occasions when her friends had gained weight and then went on quick-fix, panic diets to lose those pounds. She'd forgotten that her net weight loss was the most she had ever sustained, and that she'd felt in control in her life.

Out of the blue, Joan texted me asking my opinion on a popular fad diet and asking for a review appointment. When we met, she told me she had been enticed by the fad diet in bid to lose weight faster, but it made her feel so unwell that she couldn't sustain it. After just two days, her intuitive eating radar had kicked in and Joan very quickly realised that this was not the right thing for her body. Her internal cues were screaming at her and she couldn't ignore them. She was back on the Food Freedom track.

That whole experience taught her that the media is there to tempt and seduce you, that dieting is big business aimed at getting you hooked on a lifetime of yo-yo fads that damage your metabolic rate and self-esteem. It doesn't serve your soul or your body. At a time of vulnerability, she realised she had a choice – she could fall back to fad diets or she could focus on her goal and ask her soul to guide her.

WHAT'S THE LESSON?

When you're tempted to get your quick-fix weight loss, pause, refocus and reflect on your end goal. What did you visualise in Chapter 18? Where is your satnav programmed to take you? If you've lost sight of this, make a poster or have a symbol of it and put it in a place you see every day.

This lady made two posters with her goal written on it. She placed one at work and one at home. She wrote:

'My goal is to have and maintain a healthy body and size while living the life I love, irrespective of weight.'

Boom! I love it.

And that's how food freedom is done.

5. Children (or as I like to call them, little humans)

Little humans give you the best feedback ever.

First of all, they notice when you sit and eat with them, and they really value that time. You're nourishing yourself and feeding their beautiful souls – now that's efficient time management!

Second, they notice that you're taking your time, not rushing the meal. They may be a little resistant to turning the screens off at first, but they soon realise that they get undivided mummy or daddy time instead. It's a trade-off they would much rather have.

Third, they notice that they're not being forced to overeat. There are now clear rules on how, what and when they can eat, and children love clear messages because they know where they stand.

Fourth, they notice that their food has become a lot more colourful, and when they eat those foods they enjoy the taste and feel better. And it must be good for you because mummy/daddy is eating them daily, too!

Soon, over a relatively short space of time, the battles with getting your children to eat at the table, with no screens, including fruit and veg, no longer exist. They choose to drink water because you do. They eat veg because you do. It becomes normal for them to sit at the table and eat slowly because you do. It becomes normal to eat exactly the right portion for their needs because you do. And it becomes normal for them to snack on fruit instead of biscuits because you do. Life around food becomes less complicated, much healthier and aligned to nurturing growing humans.

The greatest feedback you can have with Food Freedom is watching and feeling the ripple effect on your children as they grow in a world free from food noise. You become the best role model of Food Freedom, and you know your work (and mine) is done when your child has the most amazing relationship with food. What a gift, my friend – what a gift!

CHAPTER TWENTY-ONE

WITH GRATITUDE

You're possibly thinking 'Why gratitude? Why should I be grateful for the curse of a fat body? A body that doesn't seem fit for me or my purpose?'

Well, it starts and ends with self-love. Be grateful right **NOW**. Love it right **NOW**. Respect it right **NOW**. Notice the things you love right **NOW**.

That body is yours to keep, love and cherish. Its appearance is based on how you respect it. If you love and respect it, it will appear loved and respected. It will show its true self. Be grateful for the perfect vehicle you have been gifted. Love every aspect of it and be grateful for its true inner beauty, and it will bring you back home. Be in love with you and the rest will shine. Shine bright, ladies and gents, shine bright!

A gift I offer my patients is a daily ritual where you

look at yourself in the mirror and notice three things you love about your body. Look at different things each day and say out loud with absolute conviction:

I love my...

I love my...

I love my...

Thank you. Thank you . Thank you

If, when you start, you struggle to think of three things, remember things that other people love or say about you. The key to this is saying 'I love' with such passion that you emotionally connect with the words. This helps you love yourself and be grateful for yourself.

The second thing I ask my patients to do is note down three things you achieve each day that are worth celebrating. They can be little or big – the key is to feel proud when you write them down, because the process becomes a celebration. Then, at moments when you're feeling down, you can read them again and remember how amazing you are, inside and out. Simply beautiful!

I'm also ending this book with gratitude for two

more reasons. First of all, because I'm grateful for your time and support in reading and taking action. Secondly, because I'm grateful that the universe has given me this gift of communicating the message of Food Freedom. For the journey I've been on and continue to follow. For the privilege of being able to support, guide, learn and prevent food noise from growing in the next generation. I thank all my patients for every lesson I've learned while facilitating their journey to Food Freedom, and for trusting the process and taking that leap of faith.

Are you ready to take that leap?
Love, trust and jump!
With much love and devotion,

Dimple x

PS – If this book saves a single life from an eating disorder and, via the charitable donations of profits, feeds several families in the process – then my work here is done!

Amen

WHERE TO GO FROM HERE...

Firstly, thank you so much for taking the time to read this book. I do not take your valued time for granted. I wanted to give you a place to go to for further support or if you are like me and want to know more. So I thought I would make it easy and save you googling. (Or you can google me if you like.)

If you would like more information or want to join my Food Freedom Facebook group where I give free help and support or would like have regular updates from my webpage then you can find me online here:

Follow me:
@nutritionwithdimple on Instagram and Facebook for recipes, tips, and more.

Visit nutritionwithdimple.com for more information about the Food Freedom Programme.

My purpose in life is to serve and benefit others by transforming your relationships to help and support the most amazing life for you! God bless and I hope to connect with you soon. X

BIBLIOGRAPHY

Bacon, L. and Aphramor, L., 'Weight Science: Evaluating the Evidence for a Paradigm Shift', *Nutrition Journal,* vol. 10, issue 9, 2011, https://nutritionj.biomedcentral.com/articles/10.1186/1475-2891-10-9.

Benefer, M.D., et al., 'Water intake and post-exercise cognitive performance: an observational study of long-distance walkers and runners', *European Journal of Nutrition*, vol. 52, issue 2, 2013, https://www.ncbi.nlm.nih.gov/pubmed/22576040.

Canfield, Jack, *The Success Principles*, 2005.

Cian, C., et al., 'Effects of fluid ingestion on cognitive function after heat stress or exercise-induced dehydration', *International Journal of Psychophysiology*, vol. 42, issue 3, November 2001, http://www.sciencedirect.com/science/article/pii/S0167876001001428.

Cleo, G., et al., 'Could habits hold the key to weight loss maintenance? A narrative review', *Journal of Human Nutrition and Dietetics*, vol. 30, issue 5, 2017, https://www.ncbi.nlm.nih.gov/pubmed/28150402.

Cortez D.N., et al., 'Evaluating the effectiveness of an empowerment program for self-care in type 2 diabetes: a cluster randomized trial', *BMC Public Health*, vol. 17, issue 41, 2017, https://www.ncbi.nlm.nih.gov/pubmed/28061840.

Davy, B., et al., 'Water Consumption Reduces Energy Intake at a Breakfast Meal in Obese Older Adults', *Journal of the American Dietetic Association*, vol. 108, issue 7, 2008, https://www.ncbi.nlm.nih.gov/pubmed/18589036.

Dennis, E.A., et al., 'Water consumption increases weight loss during a hypocaloric diet intervention in middle-aged and older adults', *Obesity (Silver Spring)*, vol. 18, issue 2, 2010, https://www.ncbi.nlm.nih.gov/pubmed/19661958.

Dulloo, A.G. and Montani, J.P., 'Pathways from dieting to weight regain, to obesity and to the metabolic syndrome: an overview', *Obesity Reviews*, vol. 16, issue S1, February 2015, https://www.ncbi.nlm.nih.gov/pubmed/25614198.

Fadda, R., et al., 'Effects of drinking supplementary water at school on cognitive performance in children', *Appetite*, vol. 59, issue. 3, December 2012, https://www.ncbi.nlm.nih.gov/pubmed/22841529.

Gaffney-Stomberg, E., et al., 'Increasing Dietary Protein Requirements in Elderly People for Optimal Muscle and Bone Health', *Journal of the American Geriatrics Society*, vol. 57, issue 6, 2009, http://onlinelibrary.wiley.com/doi/10.1111/j.1532- 5415.2009.02285.x/full.

Gotink, R.A., et al., 'Standardised Mindfulness-Based Interventions in Healthcare: An Overview of Systematic Reviews and Meta-Analyses of RCTs', *PLoS ONE*, vol. 10, issue 4, 2015, https://www.ncbi.nlm.nih.gov/pmc/articles/PMC4400080/.

Hammond, M., 'Ways Dietitians are Incorporating Mindfulness and Mindful Eating into Nutrition Counseling', *Public Health and Community Nutrition Practice Group, The Digest*, 2007.

Jackson, S.E., et al., 'Perceived weight discrimination and changes in weight, waist circumference, and weight status', *Obesity (Silver Spring)*, vol. 22, issue 12, 2014, https://www.ncbi.nlm.nih.gov/pubmed/25212272.

Lawrence, G.D., 'Dietary fats and health: dietary recommendations in the context of scientific evidence', *Advances in Nutrition*, vol. 4, May 2013, https://www.ncbi.nlm.nih.gov/pubmed/23674795.

Layman, D.K., et al., 'Dietary protein and exercise have additive effects on body composition during weight loss in adult women', *The Journal of Nutrition*, vol. 135, issue 8, August 2005, https://www.ncbi.nlm.nih.gov/pubmed/16046 715?dopt=Abstract&fref=gc.

Leahey, T., et al., 'A Cognitive-Behavioral Mindfulness Group Therapy Intervention for the Treatment of Binge Eating in Bariatric Surgery Patients', *Cognitive and Behavioral Practice*, vol. 15, 2008.

Leidy, H.J., et al., 'The role of protein in weight loss and maintenance', *The American Journal of Clinical Nutrition*, vol. 10, issue 6, June 2015, https://www.ncbi.nlm.nih.gov/ pubmed/25926512.

Longland, T.M., et al., 'Higher compared with lower dietary protein during an energy deficit combined with intense exercise promotes greater lean mass gain and fat mass loss: a randomized trial', *The American Journal of Clinical Nutrition*, vol. 103, issue 3, March 2016, https://www.ncbi.nlm.nih.gov/ pubmed/26817506.

McKenna, P., *I Can Make You Thin*, 2007, Transworld publishers

Mantzios, M. and Wilson, J.C., 'Mindfulness, Eating Behaviours, and Obesity: A Review and Reflection on Current Findings', *Current Obesity Reports*, vol. 5, issue 1, March 2015, https://www.ncbi.nlm.nih.gov/ pubmed/26627097.

Meule, A., et al., 'Enhanced behavioral inhibition in restrained eaters', *Eating Behaviors*, vol. 12, issue 2, April 2011, https://www.ncbi.nlm.nih.gov/pubmed/21385646.

Millward, D.J., 'Protein requirements and aging', *The American Journal of Clinical Nutrition*, vol. 100, issue 4, October 2014, https://www.ncbi.nlm.nih.gov/pubmed/25240087.

Morais, J.A., et al., 'Protein turnover and requirements in the healthy and frail elderly', *Journal of Nutrition Health and Aging*, vol. 11, issue 4, Jul-Aug 2006, https://www.ncbi.nlm.nih.gov/pubmed/16886097.

Murakami, K., et al., 'Association between dietary fiber, water and magnesium intake and functional constipation among young Japanese women', *European Journal of Clinical Nutrition*, vol. 61, 2007, http://www.nature.com/ejcn/journal/v61/n5/abs/1602573a.html?foxtrotcallback=true.

Polivy, J. and Herman, C.P., 'Restrained Eating and Food Cues: Recent Findings and Conclusions', *Current Obesity Reports*, vol. 6, issue 1, March 2017, https://www.ncbi.nlm.nih.gov/pubmed/28205156.

Prentice, A., et al., SACN Carbohydrates and Health Report, Public Health England, July 2015, https://www.gov.uk/government/publications/sacn-carbohydrates-and-health-report.

Pross, N., et al., 'Influence of progressive fluid restriction on mood and physiological markers of dehydration in women', *The British Journal of Nutrition*, vol. 109, issue 2, 2013, https://www.ncbi.nlm.nih.gov/pubmed/22716932.

Raja-Khan, N., et al., 'Mindfulness-Based Stress Reduction in Women with Overweight or Obesity: A Randomized Clinical Trial', *Obesity (Silver Spring)*, vol. 25, issue 8, 2017, https://www.ncbi.nlm.nih.gov/pubmed/28686006.

Riebl, S.K. and Davy, B.M., 'The Hydration Equation: Update on Water Balance and Cognitive Performance', *ACSM's Health & Fitness Journal*, vol. 17, issue 6, 2013, https://www.ncbi.nlm.nih.gov/pmc/articles/PMC4207053/.

Robson, K.M., et al., 'Development of constipation in nursing home residents', *Dis Colon Rectum*, vol. 42, issue 7, July 2000, https://www.ncbi.nlm.nih.gov/pubmed/10910239.

Ryan, P., 'Integrated Theory of Health Behavior Change', *Clinical Nurse Specialist*, vol. 23, issue 3, May-June 2009, https://www.ncbi.nlm.nih.gov/pmc/articles/PMC2778019/.

Satter, E., 'Eating competence: Nutrition Education with the Satter Eating Competence Model', *Journal of Nutrition*

Education and Behavior, vol. 39, 2007, http://www.jneb.
org/article/S1499-4046(07)00467-8/pdf.

Schvey, N.A., et al., 'The impact of weight stigma on
caloric consumption', *Obesity (Silver Spring)*, vol. 19, issue
10, 2011, https://www.ncbi.nlm.nih.gov/pubmed/21760636.

Suhr, J.A., et al., 'The relation of hydration status
to cognitive performance in healthy older adults',
International Journal of Psychophysiology, vol. 53,
issue 2, July 2004, https://www.ncbi.nlm.nih.gov/
pubmed/15210289.

Van Walleghen, E., et al., 'Pre-meal water consumption
reduces meal energy intake in older but not younger
subjects', *Obesity (Silver Spring)*, vol. 15, issue 1, 2007,
https://www.ncbi.nlm.nih.gov/pubmed/17228036.

REFERENCES

[1] As explained in *The Success Principles* by Jack Canfield.

[2] Polivy, J., 'Restrained Eating and Food Cues: Recent Findings and Conclusions', *Current Obesity Reports*.

[3] Meule, A., 'Enhanced behavioral inhibition in restrained eaters', *Eating Behaviors*.

4 Bacon, L. and Aphramor, L., 'Weight Science: Evaluating the Evidence for a Paradigm Shift', *Nutrition Journal*.

[5] According to Strohacker, et al., Stice, et al., Coakley, et al., Bild, et al., Korkeila, et al., Neumark-Sztainer, et al. and Field, et al. – as cited by Bacon, L. and Aphramor, L. in 'Weight Science: Evaluating the Evidence for a Paradigm Shift' in *Nutrition Journal*.

[6] Protein turnover and requirements in the healthy and frail elderly.
https://www.ncbi.nlm.nih.gov/pubmed/16886097

[7] Dulloo, A.G., 'Pathways from dieting to weight regain, to obesity and to the metabolic syndrome: an overview', *Obesity Reviews.*

[8] Dulloo, A.G., 'Pathways from dieting to weight regain, to obesity and to the metabolic syndrome: an overview', *Obesity Reviews.*

[9] Dulloo, A.G., 'Pathways from dieting to weight regain, to obesity and to the metabolic syndrome: an overview', *Obesity Reviews.*

[10] Bacon, L. and Aphramor, L., 'Weight Science: Evaluating the Evidence for a Paradigm Shift', *Nutrition Journal.*

[11] Bacon, L. and Aphramor, L., 'Weight Science: Evaluating the Evidence for a Paradigm Shift', *Nutrition Journal.*

[12] Bacon, L. and Aphramor, L., 'Weight Science: Evaluating the Evidence for a Paradigm Shift', *Nutrition Journal.*

[13] Dulloo, A.G., 'Pathways from dieting to weight regain, to obesity and to the metabolic syndrome: an overview',

Obesity Reviews.

[14] Schvey, N.A., 'The impact of weight stigma on caloric consumption', *Obesity (Silver Spring).*

[15] Jackson, S.E., 'Perceived weight discrimination and changes in weight, waist circumference, and weight status', *Obesity (Silver Spring).*

[16] Schvey, N.A., 'The impact of weight stigma on caloric consumption', *Obesity (Silver Spring).*

[17] Cleo, G., 'Could habits hold the key to weight loss maintenance? A narrative review', *Journal of Human Nutrition and Dietetics.*

[18] Cortez D.N., 'Evaluating the effectiveness of an empowerment program for self- care in type 2 diabetes: a cluster randomized trial', *BMC Public Health.*

[19] Ryan, P., 'Integrated Theory of Health Behavior Change', *Clinical Nurse Specialist.*

[20] For examples of this research, see:

- Riebl, S.K., 'The Hydration Equation: Update on Water Balance and Cognitive Performance', *ACSM's Health & Fitness Journal.*

- Pross, N., 'Influence of progressive fluid restriction on mood and physiological markers of dehydration in women', *The British Journal of Nutrition.*

- Benefer, M.D., 'Water intake and post-exercise cognitive performance: an observational study of long-distance walkers and runners', *European Journal of Nutrition.*

- Fadda, R., 'Effects of drinking supplementary water at school on cognitive performance in children', *Appetite.*

- Cian, C., 'Effects of fluid ingestion on cognitive function after heat stress or exercise-induced dehydration', *International Journal of Psychophysiology.*

- Suhr, J.A., 'The relation of hydration status to cognitive performance in healthy older adults', *International Journal of Psychophysiology.*

- Murakami, K., 'Association between dietary fiber, water and magnesium intake and functional constipation among young Japanese women', *European Journal of Clinical Nutrition.*

- Robson, K.M., 'Development of constipation in nursing home residents', *Dis Colon Rectum.*

[21] Dennis E.A., 'Water consumption increases weight loss during a hypocaloric diet intervention in middle-aged and

older adults', *Obesity (Silver Spring)*.

[22] See the following 2 papers:

- Davy, B., 'Water Consumption Reduces Energy Intake at a Breakfast Meal in Obese Older Adults', *Journal of the American Dietetic Association.*

- Van Walleghen, E., 'Pre-meal water consumption reduces meal energy intake in older but not younger subjects', *Obesity (Silver Spring).*

[23] Prentice, A., SACN Carbohydrates and Health Report for Public Health England. 24 Prentice, A., SACN Carbohydrates and Health Report for Public Health England. 25 Leidy, H.J., 'The role of protein in weight loss and maintenance', *The American Journal of Clinical Nutrition.*

[26] See the following research:

- Leidy, H.J., 'The role of protein in weight loss and maintenance', *The American Journal of Clinical Nutrition.*

- Morais, J.A., 'Protein turnover and requirements in the healthy and frail elderly', *Journal of Nutrition Health and Aging.*

- Millward, D.J., 'Protein requirements and aging', *The*

American Journal of Clinical Nutrition.

- Longland, T.M., 'Higher compared with lower dietary protein during an energy deficit combined with intense exercise promotes greater lean mass gain and fat mass loss: a randomized trial', *The American Journal of Clinical Nutrition.*

- Gaffney-Stomberg, E., 'Increasing Dietary Protein Requirements in Elderly People for Optimal Muscle and Bone Health', *Journal of the American Geriatrics Society.*

- Layman, D.K., 'Dietary protein and exercise have additive effects on body composition during weight loss in adult women', *The Journal of Nutrition.*

[27] Lawrence, G.D., 'Dietary fats and health: dietary recommendations in the context of scientific evidence', *Advances in Nutrition.*

[28] Satter, E., 'Eating competence: Nutrition Education with the Satter Eating Competence Model', *Journal of Nutrition Education and Behavior.*

[29] Hammond, M., 'Ways Dietitians are Incorporating Mindfulness and Mindful Eating into Nutrition Counseling', *Public Health and Community Nutrition Practice Group, The Digest.*

[30] Hammond, M., 'Ways Dietitians are Incorporating Mindfulness and Mindful Eating into Nutrition Counseling', *Public Health and Community Nutrition Practice Group, The Digest.*

[31] Mantzios, M. and Wilson, J.C., 'Mindfulness, Eating Behaviours, and Obesity: A Review and Reflection on Current Findings', *Current Obesity Reports.*

[32] Raja-Khan, N., 'Mindfulness-Based Stress Reduction in Women with Overweight or Obesity: A Randomized Clinical Trial', *Obesity (Silver Spring).*

[33] Gotink, R.A., 'Standardised Mindfulness-Based Interventions in Healthcare: An Overview of Systematic Reviews and Meta-Analyses of RCTs', *PLoS ONE.*

[34] Leahey, T., 'A Cognitive-Behavioral Mindfulness Group Therapy Intervention for the Treatment of Binge Eating in Bariatric Surgery Patients', *Cognitive and Behavioral Practice.*

[35] McKenna, P., I Can Make You Thin, 2007, *Transworld publishers Ltd.*

[36] Canfield, J., *The Success Principles.* https://www.gov.uk/government/uploads/system/uploads/attachment_data/file/61353 2/obes-phys-acti-diet-eng-2017-rep.pdf

APPENDIX

I thought it would be useful to provide a snap shot of the foods that you would include in each food group just in case you are a little confused or just need some extra guidance on what foods are included in each food group.

Before I do just be aware that most foods contain more than one food group like bread does contain some protein or pulses or legumes to contain some carbohydrates as well. I have put the foods in each group as it is seen as a high source of that nutrient. For example.

Bread contains more carbohydrate than protein therefore it is classed as a food that provides carbohydrates. So use the information as a guide.

PROTEIN FOODS

- Meat – all meats Fish and all shell fish Eggs
- Dairy – all cow's milk based i.e. cheese, yogurt, Tofu
- Pulses/legumes/beans seeds
- Vegetarian meat substitutes like Quorn

CARBOHYDRATES (COMPLEX)

- Bread – ideally wholewheat/seeded/wholemeal
- Rice
- Pasta
- Potatoes -sweet and white Cassava/yam
- Any grain – barley, oats
- Other breads – naan, chapattis, pitta, wraps

Ideally if you can opt for the wholemeal or wholegrain or brown version of these foods then that would be optimal.

FATS

Monounsaturated fats

- Olive oil
- Rapeseed oil

Saturated fat (avoid)

- Butter
- Ghee Lard

- coconut oil
- palm oils

as well as foods made from these

- pastries
- cakes
- biscuits and other foods made from hydrogenated fats.

Unsaturated fat (alternative)

- Soft spreads including margarines – sunflower, soya, corn, linseed (flaxseed), safflower, fish oil (polyunsaturated fats)

Source: British Dietetic Association, Food Fact Sheet on Healthy Eating, 2016 https://www.bda.uk.com/ foodfacts/HealthyEating.pdf

Printed in Great Britain
by Amazon